T0254480

Fundamentals of Nursing and Midwifery Research

This book presents a unique approach to teaching the principles of health research using practical case studies with which nurses and midwives can engage to gain the skills to read and understand reports, evaluate the quality of research, synthesise different studies and be able to evaluate their effectiveness when applied to clinical practice.

The book covers core concepts and principles, including the following:

- What evidence is and why understanding research is vital
- Finding reliable sources of evidence
- The nature of the research process
- Understanding quantitative and qualitative research
- Ethical considerations
- Using research to guide clinical practice

Throughout the book, activities, summaries and review questions help ground theory in real-life scenarios, showing how evidence-based practice can be applied in every aspect of nursing and midwifery care. It is designed for nurses and midwives, from those just beginning their studies to qualified practitioners undertaking their first research projects.

Lisa McKenna is Professor and Dean in the School of Nursing and Midwifery, La Trobe University, Melbourne. She has researched widely, particularly in the areas of nursing, midwifery and health professional education and workforce, and published over 250 refereed peer-reviewed journal articles along with a number of textbooks. Lisa's research expertise incorporates a range of methodologies, including quantitative, qualitative and mixed methods.

Beverley Copnell is Associate Professor in the School of Nursing and Midwifery, La Trobe University, Melbourne. Before entering academia, she worked in paediatric intensive care, a field in which she maintains an active interest. She is a member of the editorial board of *Pediatric Critical Care Medicine* and an editor of *Collegian: The Australian Journal of Nursing Practice, Scholarship and Research*. She has a long-standing interest in promoting research and evidence-based practice in nursing.

Fundamentals of Nursing and Midwifery Research

A Practical Guide for
Evidence-based Practice

Second Edition

Lisa McKenna and Beverley Copnell

Routledge
Taylor & Francis Group

LONDON AND NEW YORK

Designed cover image: Routledge

Second edition published 2024
by Routledge
4 Park Square, Milton Park, Abingdon, Oxon, OX14 4RN

and by Routledge
605 Third Avenue, New York, NY 10158

Routledge is an imprint of the Taylor & Francis Group, an informa business

© 2024 Lisa McKenna and Beverley Copnell

The right of Lisa McKenna and Beverley Copnell to be identified as authors of this work has been asserted in accordance with sections 77 and 78 of the Copyright, Designs and Patents Act 1988.

All rights reserved. No part of this book may be reprinted or reproduced or utilised in any form or by any electronic, mechanical, or other means, now known or hereafter invented, including photocopying and recording, or in any information storage or retrieval system, without permission in writing from the publishers.

Trademark notice: Product or corporate names may be trademarks or registered trademarks, and are used only for identification and explanation without intent to infringe.

First edition published by Allen & Unwin 2019

British Library Cataloguing-in-Publication Data
A catalogue record for this book is available from the British Library

Library of Congress Cataloging-in-Publication Data
Names: McKenna, Lisa, author. | Copnell, Beverley, author.
Title: Fundamentals of nursing and midwifery research: a practical guide for evidence-based practice / Lisa McKenna and Beverley Copnell.
Description: Second edition. | Abingdon, Oxon; New York, NY: Routledge, 2024. | Revised edition of: Fundamentals of nursing and midwifery research / Lisa McKenna, Beverley Copnell. 2019. | Includes bibliographical references and index.
Identifiers: LCCN 2023038426 | ISBN 9781032539546 (hbk) |
ISBN 9781032539539 (pbk) | ISBN 9781003414476 (ebk)
Subjects: LCSH: Nursing—Research. | Midwifery—Research. | Evidence-based nursing. | Medical research personnel.
Classification: LCC RT81.5 .M37 2024 | DDC 610.73072—dc23/eng/20231115
LC record available at https://lccn.loc.gov/2023038426

ISBN: 978-1-032-53954-6 (hbk)
ISBN: 978-1-032-53953-9 (pbk)
ISBN: 978-1-003-41447-6 (ebk)

DOI: 10.4324/9781003414476

Typeset in Sabon
by codeMantra

Contents

List of figures and tables   *vii*
List of boxes   *viii*
Outline of the book   *xi*
Preface   *xiii*

SECTION 1
How Do I Find and Use Evidence?   1

1 What is evidence and why do I need to understand research?   2

2 Locating evidence   13

SECTION 2
How Can I Make Sense of Research Evidence?   25

3 Understanding how research is done   26

4 Understanding quantitative research approaches   40

5 Understanding qualitative research approaches   61

SECTION 3
How Do I Critically Evaluate Research Studies?   77

6 Critiquing research   78

7 Ethics and research in nursing and midwifery   97

SECTION 4
How Do I Use Evidence to Inform My Practice?   111

  8 Applying evidence in practice   112

  9 Writing effective reviews of literature   125

10 Sharing research   135

SECTION 5
How Do I Pursue a Nursing or Midwifery Research Future?   147

11 Research pathways for nurses and midwives   148

     Glossary of terms   *165*
     Index   *173*

Figures and tables

Figures

1.1   Hierarchy of evidence   8
4.1   A normal distribution   52
4.2   Skewed distributions: (a) positive skew, (b) negative skew   52
6.1   Flow chart of a search   90

Tables

1.1   Examples of professional standards for evidence-based
      practice and research   5
2.1   Information sources and their usefulness and credibility as sources of
      research evidence   15
2.2   Results of searches conducted in MEDLINE concerning barriers to
      handwashing in nurses   20
3.1   Differences between quantitative and qualitative research approaches   29
4.1   Comparison of quantitative designs   42
4.2   Descriptive statistics and when to use them   54
10.1 Sample unstructured abstract   137
10.2 Sample structured abstract   137

Boxes

Research Examples

1.1	Hand hygiene practices	6
1.2	Barriers in evidence-based nursing practice	7
1.3	Evidence-based practice in midwifery	8
1.4	A systematic review of hand hygiene compliance (HHC)	10
2.1	Do nurses source research evidence?	20
3.1	Why do a literature review?	28
3.2	Using mixed methods to study person-centred midwifery care	31
4.1	Using a quasi-experimental design to improve person-centred care	48
4.2	Using a cross-sectional correlational design to study woman-centred midwifery care	49
4.3	Tools to measure person-centred care	57
5.1	Using qualitative descriptive research to study woman-centred midwifery care during the COVID-19 pandemic	69
5.2	Using a qualitative descriptive approach to study person-centred care	70
6.1	Vital signs trends and clinical deterioration	84
6.2	A survey to assess nursing students' vital signs monitoring	85
6.3	A nursing systematic review	91
6.4	Review of intermittent auscultation in labour	92
7.1	Ethical issues in collecting data by observation	106
7.2	Ethical issues in collecting data by survey	107
8.1	Examining evidence-based nursing and midwifery practice	116
8.2	Participatory action research in implementation of evidence-based practice	119
8.3	Realist evaluation of nursing practice	121
8.4	Realist evaluation of midwifery continuity of care	122
9.1	Scoping review of nurse fatigue and medication administration error	126
9.2	Narrative review of medications and breastfeeding	127
9.3	Systematic review of double checking to reduce medication errors	132
10.1	Increasing publication rates	143
10.2	Measuring research outputs	143
11.1	Nurse-led clinical trials	151
11.2	Midwife-led clinical trials	151
11.3	Honours degrees in Australia	152
11.4	A nursing research proposal	159

Activities

1.1	Evidence in nursing and midwifery practice	4
1.2	Evidence-based practice in nursing and midwifery	6
2.1	Searching a database	17
2.2	Constructing a strategy to search the literature	20
2.3	Levels of evidence	22
3.1	Questions suitable for quantitative and qualitative approaches	30
3.2	Differences between quantitative and qualitative research	31
3.3	Research considerations	34
3.4	Collecting research data	36
3.5	Disseminating research findings through social media	37
4.1	Comparing quantitative research designs	46
4.2	Designing a quantitative study	51
4.3	Descriptive statistics and measurement scales	55
4.4	Analysing a quantitative research paper	58
5.1	Exploring a qualitative research approach	64
5.2	Exploring person-centred care qualitatively	65
5.3	Planning qualitative research	67
5.4	Collecting qualitative data	68
5.5	Analysing a qualitative research report	73
6.1	Undertaking a research report critique	84
6.2	Using critical appraisal tools	86
6.3	Developing a systematic review protocol	88
6.4	Exploring systematic reviews	90
6.5	Developing a scoping review protocol	92
6.6	Exploring scoping reviews	92
6.7	Rapid and umbrella reviews	94
7.1	Human Research Ethics Committees	99
7.2	Risks of research	102
7.3	Informed consent	104
7.4	Clinical relationships	105
7.5	Exploring research ethics	106
7.6	Using social media sources in research	108
8.1	Responsibility for knowledge translation	113
8.2	Reflecting on knowledge translation	113
8.3	Questioning clinical practice	115
8.4	Evidence implementation	116
8.5	Exploring an evidence-based practice model	118
8.6	Participatory action research	120
8.7	Realist evaluation	121
9.1	Types of literature reviews	126
9.2	Searching for literature	129
9.3	Paraphrasing	131
9.4	Approaching a literature review	132
10.1	Think about a presentation you have given in the past	139
10.2	Now consider Alice in our case study for this chapter	139
10.3	Select three journals relevant to your area of interest	141

10.4 Again, consider Alice in our case study for this chapter   143
11.1 Exploring the clinical research nurse role   150
11.2 Exploring a research career   154
11.3 Personal reflection   154
11.4 Developing a research proposal   162

Research Tips

2.1 Useful databases for finding nursing and midwifery research articles   16
4.1 Common statistical tests and their purposes   56
4.2 Reporting standards relevant to quantitative designs   58
5.1 Common qualitative approaches used in nursing and midwifery   64
5.2 Potential data sources for qualitative research   66
6.1 Places to check for journal credibility   81
6.2 Examples of study reporting guidelines   86

Outline of the book

Section 1   How Do I Find and Use Evidence?

Chapter 1 provides an introduction to evidence in nursing and midwifery. The chapter discusses the importance of using evidence in practice and outcomes when health professionals do not use evidence to support their practice. It positions research in the context of evidence and outlines the need for nurses and midwives to be users of evidence.

Chapter 2 provides a focus on locating evidence to support nursing and midwifery practice. The chapter examines sources of research evidence along with strategies for effectively finding it and determining its credibility. It presents common databases where nursing and midwifery research can be found and strategies for conducting effective searches within them.

Section 2   How Can I Make Sense of Research Evidence?

Chapter 3 provides an overview of various steps involved in the research process. It introduces considerations in developing a research question, deciding the best approach for a research study, designing a study and identifying and accessing necessary approvals.

Chapter 4 provides an overview of quantitative research approaches commonly used in nursing and midwifery, with a focus on person-centred care. The chapter examines experimental and non-experimental research designs and processes for developing a quantitative research question. It explores different types of data, sampling procedures, data collection, basic statistical tests and the importance of validity and reliability. Finally, it discusses reporting of quantitative findings and related reporting standards.

Chapter 5 provides an overview of qualitative research approaches commonly used in nursing and midwifery, with a focus on person-centred care. The chapter explores reasons why qualitative research is popular in nursing and midwifery and introduces common approaches—namely, phenomenology, descriptive qualitative approaches and grounded theory. Using a case study, it explores steps in undertaking qualitative research, common data collection methods, sampling approaches and analysing qualitative data using thematic and content analysis. Finally, it examines considerations for ensuring the quality of qualitative research and reporting findings.

Section 3   How Do I Critically Evaluate Research Studies?

Chapter 6 provides an overview of processes for critiquing research. It introduces a step-by-step approach to evaluating research quality through questioning and critiquing tools.

Using the case example of vital signs monitoring, the chapter examines the value of nursing and midwifery research. It examines the collation of research critiques of bodies of knowledge to explore approaches to structured critical literature reviews—namely, systematic and scoping reviews—including protocol development.

Chapter 7 provides an overview of ethical considerations in nursing and midwifery research. The chapter introduces the importance of ethical approaches to research and the roles of Human Research Ethics Committees and presents the fundamental principles that should underpin all research involving human participants: research merit and integrity, beneficence and non-maleficence, respect for persons and justice. Finally, the chapter explores ethical issues arising in the emerging use of the internet and social media as data sources in research.

Section 4   How Do I Use Research Evidence to Inform My Practice?

Chapter 8 provides an overview of approaches to applying research evidence to nursing and midwifery practice. The chapter introduces the concept of knowledge translation and the questioning of clinical practice. It presents clinical practice guidelines and clinical audits as sources of practice evidence. The chapter examines some common evidence-based practice models used in health care. Finally, it explores evaluation of evidence implementation using action research and realist evaluation as sample approaches.

Chapter 9 is dedicated to the writing of effective reviews of the literature. The chapter begins by defining what a literature review seeks to achieve, types of literature reviews and the process of writing a review. It introduces a range of academic concepts important to students needing to undertake reviews of literature for academic assessments as well as for clinical work.

Chapter 10 examines the dissemination of research findings, focusing on presentations and writing for publication. It also explores strategies for increasing impact of research.

Section 5   How Do I Pursue a Nursing or Midwifery Research Future?

Chapter 11 provides insights into research career pathways available to nurses and midwives. It introduces different types of research roles common to these professions and education pathways to research careers. It explores the growing involvement of nurses and midwives in clinical trials. The second half of the chapter focuses on seeking funding for research activities and developing effective proposals for grant funding or academic work.

Preface

In today's contemporary healthcare system, research plays a major role in directing the best approaches to clinical care and practice. This is no different for the disciplines of nursing and midwifery, where increasingly there is an onus to provide the most effective care, informed by quality and current research findings. Consumers of health care, too, are much better informed than they have been in the past. With access to endless online information resources, they expect the highest levels of treatments and care. Thus, the concept of evidence-based care has to become central to the practice of nurses and midwives.

Over past decades, nurses and midwives have cared for patients based upon traditional knowledge and practices. Many have continued to practise in the ways they were originally taught in their pre-registration courses. However, this is no longer appropriate. Nurses and midwives have a professional responsibility to keep up-to-date with current research impacting on their clinical practice. This occurs in a context where there is increasing emphasis on research and rapid growth in the production of research by nurses, midwives and other health professionals. Nurses and midwives require the skills and knowledge to read and understand research reports, evaluate the quality of the research, synthesise different research studies, apply the most appropriate findings to their clinical practice and evaluate their effectiveness. Furthermore, many nurses and midwives desire to contribute directly to the production of relevant research, requiring skills in performing quality research studies relevant to their practice.

We have written this text to be a useful introduction to research and evidence-based practice for nursing and midwifery students and clinicians. It aims to be practical in its approach, so that it can be used across various stages of the professional's career. We hope to demystify the connection between research and practice for students and clinicians. Each chapter in the book has been written with an overarching case study, allowing introduced concepts to be applied to realistic situations and made less distant from clinical practice. These concepts have been kept simple to ensure they are relevant, even to the beginning student of nursing or midwifery. In each chapter, we have also presented examples of actual research studies that have been conducted and are relevant to the topic being covered to demonstrate examples of how these aspects have been studied. Throughout each chapter, we include a number of activities to assist the learner to work directly with concepts as they apply to their individual situation. At the end of each chapter, we have included a series of review and reflection questions to facilitate assessment of learning and understanding, as well as questions that can be used to promote discussions in research groups or class-based situations.

The text has been developed as a series of sections that aim to progressively build the reader's fundamental knowledge and skills. Section 1 consists of two chapters. Within this section, Chapter 1 introduces the concept of evidence and explains why nurses and midwives need to understand research. The chapter introduces various professional and regulatory requirements for nurses and midwives to use evidence-based practice. Chapter 2 begins to explore how and where relevant evidence can be found, facilitating skills in searching for evidence.

Section 2 is focused on making sense of research evidence. This section contains three chapters that give an overview of research and different research approaches to provide a foundation for the reader in reading and understanding a variety of types of research studies. Chapter 3 presents a detailed introduction to the research process and how one goes about doing a research study. Chapter 4 examines quantitative research approaches with an overview of types of studies and statistical tests. Chapter 5 explores a variety of qualitative approaches to research, including how they can be undertaken.

Section 3 focuses on assisting the reader to develop skills in critically reading and evaluating research that could be used to inform clinical practice. This section consists of two chapters. Chapter 6 details step-by-step approaches to evaluating the quality of research studies and their applicability to practice. Chapter 7 introduces the important area of ethics in research. It provides an overview of ethical processes and considerations underpinning the conduct of research, ensuring that the reader has the skills to evaluate whether research has been conducted ethically.

Section 4 takes the learning from previous chapters into its application through evidence-based practice. This section consists of two chapters. Chapter 8 examines the concept of knowledge translation and how evidence can be taken from published research into guiding clinical practice. The important aspect of evaluating the application of research evidence to practice is detailed in this chapter. Chapter 9 builds on previous chapters to examine how research can be synthesised into different types of literature reviews to inform and guide practice, while Chapter 10 covers strategies for sharing research outcomes.

In a context where nurses and midwives are increasingly engaging in research activity, the final section, consisting of one chapter, explores potential research career pathways. Chapter 11 examines the nurse or midwife as evidence generator as well as research roles that nurses and midwives assume. The chapter examines available educational pathways that can be taken to further develop research expertise. Increasingly, nurses and midwives are expected to write proposals for research, whether for educational purposes or when seeking funding to support their research ideas. The chapter concludes with a step-by-step overview of how to go about writing an effective research proposal and suggests avenues that can be pursued for seeking funding to support research.

We hope that students and clinicians alike will find this text to be a valuable resource, assisting them to understand research and its application to clinical nursing and midwifery practice and contributing to the delivery of up-to-date and relevant evidence-informed optimal care.

Lisa McKenna
Beverley Copnell

Section 1

How Do I Find and Use Evidence?

Evidence-based practice is a key requirement of the work of nurses and midwives. It is often mandated as a part of professional practice standards and works to ensure the care delivered to patients is based on research proving its effectiveness. It is not considered appropriate for nurses and midwives to continue to practise in the same way throughout their careers; rather, practice needs to develop according to new and emerging research. Furthermore, today's healthcare consumers are more educated than in past decades. Through online resources, people have ready access to up-to-date research findings and are more informed about their conditions and expectations of care. This increases the requirement for nurses and midwives to be abreast of current evidence relevant to their daily practice.

This section is dedicated to the area of evidence for nursing and midwifery practice and examines professional requirements for incorporating evidence into practice. Through a particular focus on hand hygiene, the section examines what constitutes evidence, locating appropriate evidence and evidence appraisal.

Chapter 1 introduces the concept of evidence and why it is important for nursing and midwifery. It explores what it means to be a user of evidence and introduces hierarchies of evidence.

Chapter 2 builds on the previous chapter to examine where and how credible evidence can be found, and the appraisal of evidence for informing practice.

DOI: 10.4324/9781003414476-1

1   What is evidence and why do I need to understand research?

Learning objectives

After working through this chapter, you should be able to:

- Discuss what is meant by *evidence* in nursing and midwifery
- Outline the importance of evidence for health professional practice
- Discuss the relationship between evidence and research in nursing and midwifery
- Identify the role of the nurse or midwife as a user of evidence
- Define the term *evidence-based practice*
- Identify sources of good evidence
- Outline professional requirements for nurses and midwives in relation to evidence-based practice
- Define the term *systematic review*

Key terms and concepts

Data analysis, data collection, dissemination, evidence, evidence-based practice, hierarchy of evidence, hypothesis, literature review, practice guidelines, research, research process, research question, quality patient care, systematic review.

Case study overview

Effective handwashing is an important, and sometimes underestimated, task of health professionals that has the potential to directly impact on the wellbeing of patients. If micro-organisms are allowed to move from person to person through poor handwashing, this can result in serious nosocomial (hospital-acquired) infections, which may require prolonged hospitalisation or even lead to unanticipated deaths. Effective handwashing is, therefore, fundamentally important. However, varying advice exists about correct handwashing techniques and for how long handwashing should take place. In addition, hospitals provide alcohol-based disinfectants for hand sanitisation. How then do health professionals know the most effective methods of hand hygiene to reduce negative patient outcomes?

DOI: 10.4324/9781003414476-2

Introduction

Evidence-based practice is a key requirement of the work of nurses and midwives. Hence, an understanding of evidence and how it informs practice is important. This chapter introduces the concept of evidence in nursing and midwifery and how this evidence relates to practice. It also clarifies the connection between evidence and research and its importance in evidence-based nursing practice. Hierarchies of evidence are discussed, along with the role of systematic review and its benefits for nursing and midwifery.

What is evidence?

Nursing and midwifery practice is described as being underpinned by **evidence**. However, what does that mean? Using our case study about handwashing, we can begin to define it. The case study raises a question about how health professionals know the most effective methods of hand hygiene to reduce negative patient outcomes. This is where evidence comes in. Evidence in such cases relates to research findings that inform the best possible practice. Take, for example, a study conducted to compare the effectiveness of alcohol-based disinfectants with that of handwashing with soap and water in reducing the spread of different viruses. Washing hands with soap and water for 30 seconds was found to be more effective than using the alcohol-based products in removing norovirus, a virus that often causes gastroenteritis outbreaks in nursing homes (Tuladhar et al., 2015). This suggests that in some practice settings handwashing for 30 seconds with soap and water is the most effective option; hence, such evidence should guide practice.

So, going back to our original question, evidence is information, generated through research, that supports nursing and midwifery practice. In some cases, the findings from many research studies have been collated into practice guidelines that can directly inform health professionals' practice. The extent of infection acquired through hand contact led the World Health Organization to use evidence to develop its own practice guidelines for use across Australian health care. This led to the creation of the Five Moments for Hand Hygiene. Using research findings, five key moments when microorganisms can spread via hand contact in health care were identified:

1 Before patient contact
2 Before aseptic task
3 After body fluid exposure risk
4 After patient contact
5 After contact with patient surroundings (World Health Organization, 2017)

This process has been adopted widely around the world, including by the National Health Service in the United Kingdom and the Australian Commission on Safety and Quality in Health Care (2017) as part of the National Hand Hygiene Initiative to reduce nosocomial infection. As a result, it directly impacts on the practice of health professionals. Practice guidelines such as these also constitute evidence for practice, as they have been developed based upon the collation of findings of rigorous research.

What happens if health professionals do not use evidence?

Quality health care is dependent on health professionals applying current evidence to support the care they deliver to patients and communities. However, many health professionals do not adopt new practice supported by the latest evidence, choosing instead to continue with the practice they were originally taught. While that practice was probably seen to be the most effective at the time they learnt it, it may since have been disproven by research. In such cases, patients may receive inappropriate or ineffective care or may be put at increased risk of complications. If we take hand hygiene and the research by Tuladhar et al. (2015) as an example, a health professional who is carrying norovirus and washes their hands for ten seconds may carry the virus on to the next patient, who may subsequently become infected and develop gastroenteritis, which can have very serious consequences for the elderly and frail. Hence, evidence that directly informs practice can enhance patient care and health outcomes.

Activity 1.1   Evidence in nursing and midwifery practice

List the key reasons why nurses and midwives need to use evidence in practice.

Where does research fit in?

So far, we have explored the role of evidence in nursing and midwifery practice and alluded to its connection with research. However, just collecting existing research is not sufficient to implement it into practice. There is good research and not-so-good research, so it is important to understand the **research process** and to critique or evaluate the quality of the research in order to determine whether or not to use it to support practice. In this section of the chapter, we will begin to explore the research process, and we will continue to build on this in subsequent chapters.

While there are various approaches to research, all follow a consistent and systematic process:

- **Problem or issue** Generally, research is conducted to generate new knowledge to address a particular problem or examine an issue.
- **Literature review** Existing research studies are explored to see if the problem has already been addressed. If the research has already been done recently, there may be no need for new studies to be conducted. However, if there is a gap in the existing literature, it is an indication for new research to be conducted. Hence, the literature review provides the background against which a new study is developed.
- **Research question** From the problem or issue, the researcher develops a question—the research question—which the research seeks to answer. The research question should be clear, specific and able to be answered.
- **Ethical approval** If the study requires the collection of data relating to humans or animals, the researcher will be required to have the work evaluated by an ethics committee to ensure it is to be conducted in an ethical manner. The aim of ethical consideration is to confirm that the participants' rights are adhered to and participants are not put at any unnecessary risk by taking part in the research.
- **Data collection** The researcher next determines the best way, or method, in which to collect the data needed to answer the research question. This can take a number of forms—for example, questionnaires, interviews or observations.

- **Data analysis** Once all of the data are collected, the researcher analyses them to determine the research findings. This might involve mathematical calculations for numerical data or identification of patterns of words or phrases for text-based data.
- **Reporting or dissemination** Once the findings have been determined, they are made available for others to apply them. Study findings are often reported through published peer-reviewed journal articles and at professional conferences or may be presented directly in reports to governments or other organisations.

We will explore these steps in more detail in Chapter 3.

Being a user of research

Nurses and midwives are increasingly undertaking research to add to the evidence base and improve the care they deliver. However, while not all will actually undertake research, all nurses and midwives are required to use research to underpin their practice, as any other professional does. This is reinforced through professional practice standards for the disciplines, such as those outlined in Table 1.1.

Table 1.1 Examples of professional standards for evidence-based practice and research

Australia	
Registered Nurse Standards for Practice (NMBA, 2016)	"RNs use a variety of thinking strategies and the best available evidence in making decisions and providing safe, quality nursing practice within person-centred and evidence-based frameworks" The registered nurse "accesses, analyses, and uses the best available evidence, that includes research findings, for safe, quality practice" (Standard 1.1)
Midwife Standards for Practice (NMBA, 2018)	"Promotes health and wellbeing through evidence-based midwifery practice. The midwife supports women's wellbeing by providing safe, quality midwifery health care using the best available evidence and resources, with the principles of primary health care and cultural safety as foundations for practice" (Standard 1)
Enrolled Nurse Standards for Practice (NMBA, 2016)	"Provides nursing care that is informed by research evidence" (Standard 8)
New Zealand	
Competencies for Registered Nurses (Te Kaunihera Tapuhi o Aotearoa/Nursing Council of New Zealand, 2016)	"Participates in quality improvement activities to monitor and improve standards of nursing" (Competency 4.3)
Standards of Clinical & Cultural Competence & Conduct (Te Tatau o te Whare Kahu/ Midwifery Council, 2020)	"The midwife applies comprehensive theoretical and scientific knowledge with the affective and technical skills needed to provide effective and safe midwifery care" (Competency 2)
United Kingdom	
Standards of proficiency for registered nurses (NMC, 2018)	"Demonstrate an understanding of research methods, ethics and governance in order to critically analyse, safely use, share and apply research findings to promote and inform best nursing practice" (Outcome 1.7)

(Continued)

Table 1.1 (Continued)

United Kingdom	
Standards of proficiency for midwives (NMC, 2019)	"Demonstrate the knowledge, skills, and ability to identify, critically analyse, and interpret research evidence and local, national, and international data and reports" (Outcome 1.4) "Use, share and apply research findings and lessons from data and reports to promote and inform best midwifery policy and practice, and to support women's evidence-informed decision-making" (Outcome 1.5)

Activity 1.2   Evidence-based practice in nursing and midwifery

Review your local practice standards. How are evidence-based practice or research utilisation incorporated? Consider the skills that might be required.

As a student or clinician, what are your responsibilities around understanding research?

Research Example 1.1   Hand hygiene practices

Hand hygiene is fundamental to prevention of the spread of infection and it became a key focus on reducing spread of virus during the COVID-19 pandemic. In a study in one hospital in France, Huang et al. (2021) used an automated system to record healthcare workers' hand hygiene on entry and exit from patients' rooms. They identified a relationship between the available COVID-19 data and hand hygiene compliance (HHC). Overall, they found that hand hygiene on entry to rooms decreased over time. Hand hygiene on exit from patients' rooms increased by 13.73% during the first wave, decreased by 9.87% during lockdown and then increased by 2.82% again in the second wave. The researchers concluded that healthcare workers adjusted their behaviour at different times during the pandemic.

Huang, F., Armando, M., Dufau, S., Florea, O., Brouqui, P. & Boudjema, S., 2021, 'COVID-19 outbreak and healthcare worker behavioural change toward hand hygiene practice', *Journal of Hospital Infection*, vol. 111, pp. 27–34.

Questions for consideration

- What are the implications of this study's findings?
- How might health professionals use this evidence to improve care?

The standards' requirements for nurses and midwives to practise in an evidence-based way serve to ensure that patients and other health consumers receive the most effective care informed by best practice. They also serve to protect nurses and midwives, by making them accountable for their practice and the care they deliver should they be questioned about their actions in any particular situation.

As a mandated component of the roles of nurses and midwives, evidence needs to be translated directly into practice. However, research into this area suggests that it can be challenging. A cross-sectional survey (see Chapter 4) conducted by Stokke et al. (2014) in Norway with 185 nurses found that nurses held positive views about **evidence-based practice**; however, they only practised it to a small extent. This was attributed to their feeling unprepared to undertake evidence-based practice and their belief that resources to do so were limited. The researchers concluded that it was important to be educationally prepared to use evidence and that there was a need for a culture in the clinical setting to facilitate it.

Determining levels of evidence

Not all research is considered equal. Evidence elicited from some types of research is regarded as being more credible than others, and evidence sources are often ranked into a **hierarchy of evidence**. While there is some variation in how these are presented, the highest level is usually accorded to systematic reviews and meta-analyses. While we will not delve into the various types of studies in detail here, it is important to acknowledge that there are different types of evidence and that these are accorded varied levels of credibility. Overall, the higher the evidence is on the pyramid, the better its quality is and the greater the confidence we can have about its application (Figure 1.1).

Research Example 1.2   Barriers in evidence-based nursing practice

While evidence-based practice is recognised as vital for effective patient care, nurses have been slow to adopt it. Many studies have explored nurses' use of research in practice to attempt to understand why this is the case. In one study, Hendricks and Cope (2017) sought to discover whether nurses read research articles, understood them and used the findings in practice. The researchers used a survey of nurses in one hospital in Western Australia. A total of 95 nurses completed the survey. The findings indicated that the nurses found research articles difficult to understand, and 84% reported only sometimes understanding what they were reading. In addition, 64% had not taken any studies in research. This reinforces the need for nurses to have the skills to interpret research findings.

J. Hendricks & Cope, V., 2017, 'Research is not a "scary" word: Registered nurses and the barriers to research utilisation', *Nordic Journal of Nursing Research*, vol. 37, no. 1, pp. 44–50.

Questions for consideration

- Do you think the findings of this study are common to all nurses and midwives?
- What strategies could be used to develop necessary skills for reading and understanding research in nurses and midwives?

Research Example 1.3   Evidence-based practice in midwifery

Little has been written about midwives' application of research findings to their care of childbearing women. However, evidence-based practice is key to ensuring women receive the most effective and appropriate care. In one Australian study, De Leo et al. (2021) conducted research to understand the information and support that midwives needed to be able to implement evidence-based practice and hence, practice change. They interviewed eight midwife leaders using a combination of focus group and individual interviews. Findings indicated there were numerous challenges to implementing evidence-based practice including access to resources, time, as well as skills and knowledge about the process. Resources to support evidence-based practice and practice change, along with mentoring, were seen as needed. The researchers concluded that evidence-based practice was important in improving the quality of midwifery care and health outcomes for childbearing women and their newborns.

De Leo, A., Bayes, S., Butt, J., Bloxsome, D. & Geraghty, S., 2021, 'Midwifery leaders' views on the factors considered crucial to implementing evidence-based practice in clinical areas', *Women and Birth*, vol. 34, pp. 22–29.

Questions for consideration

- Do you think the findings of this study are common to all nurses and midwives?
- How might nurses and midwives manage requests for interventions that are not evidence based?

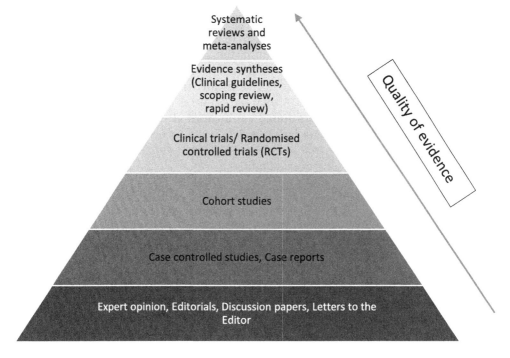

Figure 1.1 Hierarchy of evidence.

Another approach commonly used in clinical settings for determining levels of evidence is the Grading of Recommendations, Assessment, Development and Evaluation guideline. In this approach, randomised controlled trials are considered of high to moderate quality evidence, while observational studies are considered low or very quality depending on several criteria (Guyatt et al., 2011).

Systematic review

At the top of the hierarchy of evidence sits systematic review of randomised controlled trials (see Chapter 4). A **systematic review** is an analysis of a collection of individual studies on the same topic that is conducted in a structured and auditable way. In a sense, systematic reviews are research studies in their own right. These types of reviews are becoming an increasingly popular undertaking with nurses and midwives. One reason for this is that they collate the findings of smaller research studies to draw larger conclusions, and much of the research conducted by nurses and midwives is small and local in nature, unlike that in other scientific disciplines. Often, systematic reviews are also used to identify gaps in existing knowledge, to guide development of new studies.

Similar to a research study, a systematic review is underpinned by a specific question or aim. To demonstrate, we will examine a systematic review conducted by Doronina et al. (2017) that sought to explore the effectiveness of strategies to increase HHC of nurses in the hospital setting. The researchers wanted to identify frequently used interventions that specifically improved compliance and hand hygiene behaviour.

The next step in systematic review is to develop a **protocol** (outline) defining the boundaries and inclusion criteria for the review—for example, which databases will be searched, the timeframe from which papers will be included, the type of study design that will be used, the population that will be studied and the keywords and phrases that will be used to undertake the search for relevant studies. Doronina et al. (2017) included trials (see Chapter 4) from 2014 to 2017, as a previous review had included studies up to 2014. They searched a number of databases, including MEDLINE, Embase, CINAHL and Cochrane. From this, the researchers identified 303 studies as potentially meeting their inclusion criteria and on closer examination identified six to be included for analysis. A key aspect of systematic review is assessment of the quality of each study according to set evaluation criteria.

Once the final papers for inclusion have been determined, they can be grouped for analysis. Examination of the final six papers used in the review by Doronina et al. (2017) identified that multimodal, single-component and dual interventions were all able to improve hand hygiene compliance. They also concluded that higher rates and longer sustainability were enhanced with more than one intervention and the strategy was led by team leaders or managers. These findings have the potential to inform managers and organisations seeking to promote high hand hygiene compliance and influence educators developing programs for improving compliance.

Chapter summary

Evidence is fundamental to effective nursing and midwifery practice. This chapter has introduced the concept of evidence and the importance of reliable evidence for quality care delivery. The relationship between evidence and research has been discussed,

---

Research Example 1.4   A systematic review of hand hygiene compliance (HHC)

In 2022, Mouajou et al. published a systematic review of 35 research studies. They wanted to determine an optimal threshold for HHC among healthcare workers in preventing hospital-acquired infections. They found that most studies reported HHC to be between 60% and 70% and concluded that most hospital-acquired infection rates could be achieved at approximately 60%. However, they also concluded that the quality of available evidence was low, there was a lack of raw data, and differences in data meant that detailed statistical analysis was not possible.

Mouajou, V., Adams, K., DeLisle, G. & Quach, C., 2022, 'Hand hygiene compliance in the prevention of hospital-acquired infections: A systematic review', *Journal of Hospital Infection*, vol. *119*, pp. 33–48.

---

along with an overview of the research process. The responsibility of nurses and midwives to be research utilisers has been considered. Finally, hierarchies of evidence have been introduced, with a focus on systematic review. In the next chapter, we will build on this work to examine processes for finding suitable evidence and assessing its quality.

Questions for consideration

- What is the benefit of collating studies in a systematic review?
- How might nurses and midwives put these findings into practice?
- What cautions should be applied to the application of findings to practice?

Chapter review questions

- What is meant by *evidence* in nursing and midwifery practice?
- What is the relationship between evidence and research?
- What professional requirements impact on nurses' and midwives' use of evidence in practice?
- What are the key steps in the research process?
- What constitutes a systematic review?

Questions for discussion

- Why is evidence important for nursing, midwifery and health professional practice?
- How can nurses and midwives contribute to research knowledge and use?
- What are some of the challenges nurses and midwives face in utilising evidence in practice?
- What strategies could be used to promote evidence application in nursing and midwifery practice?

Questions for personal reflection

_____

- What are your personal expectations of healthcare providers with regard to being abreast of current evidence in their field?
- What strategies can you employ to build your understanding of evidence and research in your own profession?
- How do you see your own professional responsibilities with regard to evidence-based practice?

Useful web resources

Australian Nursing and Midwifery Federation (2019) Nursing and Midwifery Research Policy <https://www.anmf.org.au/media/5fjnxxhu/p_nursing_midwifery_research.pdf>.
Health Research Council New Zealand (2023) <https://www.hrc.govt.nz/>.
Medical Research Council (United Kingdom) (2023) <https://www.ukri.org/councils/mrc/>.
National Health and Medical Research Council (2023) Research Policy <https://www.nhmrc.gov.au/research-policy>.
National Institute of Nursing Research (United States) (2023) <www.ninr.nih.gov>.
Singapore Clinical Research Institute (2023) <https://www.scri.edu.sg/>.

References and further reading

Australian Commission on Safety and Quality in Health Care, 2017, *National Hand Hygiene Initiative*, <www.safetyandquality.gov.au/our-work/healthcare-associated-infection/hand-hygiene/>.
Castle, N., Handler, S. & Wagner, L., 2016, 'Hand hygiene practices reported by nurse aides in nursing homes', *Journal of Applied Gerontology*, vol. 35, no. 3, pp. 267–285.
Doronina, O., Jones, D., Martello, M., Biron, A. & Lavoie-Tremblay, M., 2017, 'A systematic review on the effectiveness of interventions to improve hand hygiene compliance of nurses in the hospital setting', *Journal of Nursing Scholarship*, vol. 49, no. 2, pp. 143–152.
Guyatt, G., Oxman, A.D., Akl, E.A., Kunz, R., Vist, G., Brozek, J., Norris, S., Falck-Ytter, Y., Glasziou, P., DeBeer, H., Jaeschke, R., Rind, D., Meerpohl, J., Dahm, P. & Schünemann, H.J., 2011, 'GrADE guidelines: 1. Introduction – GRADE evidence profiles and summary of findings tables', *Journal of Clinical Epidemiology*, vol. 64, pp. 383–394.
Hendricks, J. & Cope, V., 2017, 'Research is not a "scary" word: Registered nurses and the barriers to research utilisation', *Nordic Journal of Nursing Research*, vol. 37, no. 1, pp. 44–50.
Huang, F., Armando, M., Dufau, S., Florea, O., Brouqui, P. & Boudjema, S., 2021, 'COVID-19 outbreak and healthcare worker behavioural change toward hand hygiene practice', *Journal of Hospital Infection*, vol. 111, pp. 27–34.
Kennedy, H.P., Doig, E., Hackley, B. & Leslie, M.S., 2012, '"The midwifery two-step": A study on evidence-based midwifery practice', *Journal of Midwifery and Women's Health*, vol. 57, pp. 454–460.
Luangasanatip, N., Hongsuwan, M., Limmathurotsakul, D., Lubell, Y., Lee, A.S., Harbarth, S., Day, N.P.J., Graves, N. & Cooper, B.S., 2015, 'Comparative efficacy of interventions to promote hand hygiene in hospital: Systematic review and network meta-analysis', *British Medical Journal*, vol. 351, article **h3728**.
Mouajou, V., Adams, K., DeLisle, G. & Quach, C., 2022, 'Hand hygiene compliance in the prevention of hospital-acquired infections: A systematic review', *Journal of Hospital Infection*, vol. 119, pp. 33–48.
National Health and Medical Research Council, 2009, *NHMRC Levels of Evidence and Grades for Recommendations for Developers of Guidelines*, <https://www.nhmrc.gov.au/sites/default/files/images/NHMRC%20Levels%20and%20Grades%20(2009).**pdf**>.

Nursing and Midwifery Board of Australia, 2016, *Registered Nurse Standards for Practice*, Melbourne: NMBA.

Nursing and Midwifery Board of Australia, 2018, *Midwife Standards for Practice*, Melbourne: NMBA.

Nursing and Midwifery Council, 2018, *Future Nurse: Standards of Proficiency for Registered Nurses*, London: NMC.

Nursing and Midwifery Council, 2019, *Standards of Proficiency for Midwives*, London: NMC.

Stokke, K., Olsen, N.R., Espehaug, B. & Nortvedt, M.W., 2014, 'Evidence based practice beliefs and implementation among nurses: A cross-sectional study', *BMC Nursing*, vol. *13*, no. 8, <www.biomedcentral.com/1472-6955/13/8>.

Te Kaunihera Tapuhi o Aotearoa/Nursing Council of New Zealand, 2016, *Competencies for Registered Nurses*, New Zealand.

Te Tatau o te Whare Kahu/Midwifery Council, 2020, *Standards of Clinical & Cultural Competence & Conduct*, New Zealand.

Tuladhar, E., Hazeleger, W.C., Koopmans, M., Zwietering, M.H., Duizer, H. & Beumer, R.R., 2015, 'Reducing viral contamination from finger pads: Handwashing is more effective than alcohol-based hand disinfectants', *Journal of Hospital Infection*, vol. *90*, no. 3, pp. 226–234.

World Health Organization, 2017, *Five Moments for Hand Hygiene*, <http://who.int/gpsc/tools/Five_moments/en/>.

2 Locating evidence

Learning objectives

After working through this chapter, you should be able to:

- Discuss different types of evidence used to support nursing and midwifery practice
- Identify credible sources of evidence
- Search for and locate appropriate literature to help answer a clinical question
- Utilise a variety of academic databases containing nursing and midwifery research
- Construct effective evidence searching strategies
- Differentiate between levels of evidence in various types of research

Key terms and concepts

Boolean operator, databases, evidence, evidence hierarchies, journals, keywords, levels of evidence, Medical Subject Headings, MeSH terms, truncator, wildcard.

Case study overview

For a university assignment, Yasmin is required to find and summarise evidence on a particular aspect of handwashing. The assignment instructions state that the evidence must be no more than five years old and must be relevant to nurses. Students can choose which aspect they focus on. Yasmin decides to look at barriers to handwashing.

Chapter introduction

The previous chapter introduced the concept of evidence-based practice and its importance in nursing. Evidence in this context is defined as knowledge derived from systematic research. This chapter examines sources of existing research evidence and describes how to undertake a search for evidence. Evidence hierarchies, introduced in the previous chapter, are explored in more detail.

Where can I find evidence?

When we talk about looking for information, whether for an assignment, a literature review or any other reason, it is important to distinguish between research evidence and other types of information that are not derived from research. The latter may be useful

DOI: 10.4324/9781003414476-3

(for instance, in providing background or contextual information) but do not directly address the specific topic or question. Finding evidence means finding reports of completed research. While there is a wide range of sources of general information, not all of these are useful in locating evidence.

The most useful source of reported research is academic journals, in which research is published in the form of articles, or papers. Journals may be discipline specific (for example, nursing, midwifery, medical or allied health disciplines), speciality specific (for example, paediatric, mental health or oncology) or both. Not all journals are of a similar quality; in Chapter 6, we will look at how to evaluate a journal to assist in deciding how credible the evidence is. Research published in reputable journals has been subjected to a process called **peer review**, which means it has been evaluated by at least two people who are likely to have expertise in the area of research, the methods used or both. The article will have been through a number of changes before the reviewers and the editor of the journal were confident that it was fit to publish. Sometimes very large studies are published in book form because there is too much information to fit in to the confines of a journal article. The book will usually have undergone a review of some kind, but the process may not be clear to a reader. Textbooks, a common source of information for student assignments, are unlikely to contain research reports, although they may include references to research, which can be used to find original reports. However, as textbooks take some time to write and publish, the references may not reflect the latest research findings.

Research reports can sometimes be found outside academic sources, in which case they are said to be **grey literature**. There are several reasons why research findings may not be published in journals or books. The research may have been completed very recently and the researchers have only presented it at a conference, in which case the abstract (or sometimes the whole presentation) will have been published in the conference proceedings. The research may have been undertaken by government or other institutions and disseminated only as a standalone report. It may have been carried out as part of a university higher degree and written up only as a thesis. These types of research reports may not have been subjected to the same scrutiny as academic journal articles, and therefore their credibility can be questionable.

Table 2.1 lists commonly used sources of information, their usefulness in terms of locating research evidence and their credibility. Academic journals are the best and most useful sources of research evidence. However, journals publish several types of articles in addition to research reports—for instance, editorials, letters, and discussion and opinion pieces. These kinds of articles are not considered evidence; therefore, it is important to be able to recognise the different categories. Many journals actually indicate the category within the article itself, so this is the first thing to look for. Reports of research studies are characterised by the following:

- They usually include the word *research* or *study* somewhere in the abstract or in the early part of the article.
- They give a clearly expressed aim, usually at the end of the introduction section, which makes it clear that the article is reporting on a research study.
- They include a section labelled 'Methods' or 'Methodology', and the study design (see Section 2) should be obvious. Many journals, but not all, insist that the design is specified in the article title.
- They have a section called 'Results' or 'Findings'.

Table 2.1 Information sources and their usefulness and credibility as sources of research evidence

Source	Availability of evidence	Accessibility of evidence	Credibility
Journals	The commonest location	Easy to find	High
Books	Relatively rare	Can be difficult to find	Probably good; may not be clear
Textbooks	Unlikely to find	N/A	Probably good; may not be clear
Theses	Common location	Can be difficult to find	Unclear
Websites	Sometimes can be found	Full report may not be available	Unclear; not recommended except in specific circumstances
Mass media, social media	Findings may be mentioned	Full report not available	Unclear; locate original source

Another type of article, which may have a similar format to that listed above, is a **literature review**, which brings together some or all of the literature on a particular topic. There are different kinds of review articles; we will look at these in detail in Chapters 8 and 9. They can be useful when beginning to explore a topic, as they can help clarify ideas, they quickly give an overview of the sort of research that has been done on the topic, and their reference lists can help to find original research reports. However, they are not usually considered evidence in themselves. An exception is a specific type of literature review called a *systematic review* (introduced in Chapter 1), which is carried out using a highly rigorous process and aims to reanalyse the findings of the included studies. Literature review articles should be identified as such in the title, the abstract or both.

How do I find evidence?

Although some print versions are produced, most journals nowadays are published online, which simplifies finding and retrieving their content. However, it is neither efficient nor effective to attempt to find literature by using a generic search engine, such as Google. First, search engines do not have the ability to perform complex search procedures that eliminate irrelevant material at the same time as finding relevant material that may use slightly different terminology from your search term. Second, as most journals require a subscription, you will be unable to retrieve most of the articles you find in this way. Lastly, it can be very difficult for inexperienced researchers to discern the quality of the results returned by search engines.

Journal articles can be found using a specifically targeted search engine such as Google Scholar, and you can be more confident in the quality of the material found by this type of search engine. However, the other limitations still apply. Usually, these search engines are used only in specific circumstances (for example, when undertaking a systematic review; see Chapter 6) to ensure no articles have been missed.

The best way to find research evidence is by searching a database—an electronic catalogue, or index. When you search a database, you are not searching the internet. There are hundreds of commercially available databases (and a few that are publicly available) that can be accessed through hospital and university libraries. Most databases are discipline specific, indexing material from journals relevant to one or more professions or to a subject area. (Research tip 2.1 lists some of the databases that collate nursing and midwifery journal articles.) It is important to note that even within a specific discipline, not all relevant journals are indexed in any one database. A thorough search for available evidence includes searching a number of databases to ensure nothing has been missed. Hospital and university libraries also usually have a searchable catalogue that contains all the material that they hold or subscribe to. Searching the catalogue can prove useful for finding assignment information, but catalogues also have their drawbacks, the main one being that they are only available to employees or students of the particular institution, and therefore the search cannot be replicated by anyone outside. This is important if you need to show exactly how you obtained the material.

Let us now turn to our case study and consider the steps involved in searching a database. Yasmin has decided to use MEDLINE to search for evidence on barriers to nurses washing their hands. Note that at this stage Yasmin's topic is expressed as a phrase, rather than as a question. If you do not know very much about a topic and what sort of research has been done on it, this is a good way to start. If Yasmin found that there was a great deal of literature on her topic, she could then refine it; for instance, she might decide to concentrate on strategies to overcome barriers, or, if there was a lot of literature, to look at whether one specific strategy was effective. For now, we will stick with the broader topic.

If Yasmin searched using the phrase *"barriers to nurses washing their hands"*, the database would attempt to find that exact phrase. While it may have been used in some articles, it is almost certain that variations on the wording would also have been used, and these articles would not be found. The first step, then, is to identify the key concepts in the topic—these are called **search terms**. In Yasmin's case, the search terms are *handwashing*, *barriers* and *nurses*. In this example, the key concepts are easy to identify; if the problem or issue driving the search is more complex, and especially if a structured literature review is being conducted, the concepts should be determined using the mnemonic 'PICO', which stands for Population/Problem, Intervention, Comparator and Outcome (Aromataris & Riitano, 2014). We will discuss this in more detail in Chapter 6.

There are a number of ways to perform a search using the identified search terms. One way is to enter these terms directly into the database's search function—this is called **keyword searching**. In this strategy, the database will search for the term exactly as it is

---

Research Tip 2.1   Useful databases for finding nursing and midwifery research articles

Cochrane Library	Systematic reviews and meta-analyses
CINAHL	Cumulative Index to Nursing and Allied Health Literature
DOAJ	Directory of Open Access Journals
EMBASE	Biomedical literature
ERIC	Educational Resources Information Center; useful for finding articles related to nursing and midwifery education
Joanna Briggs Institute	Best-practice information and systematic reviews
MEDLINE	Medical, nursing and allied health literature (closely related to PubMed)
MIDIRS	Maternity and infant care
Proquest	Nursing and allied health database
PsycINFO	Psychology and mental health
PubMed	Medical and allied health literature

entered. However, these exact terms may not have been used in all relevant articles, so it is important to think of potential synonyms. For instance, rather than *barriers*, some authors may have used the term *obstacles*.

To include all of the relevant concepts in the search, the keywords have to be combined. This can be done in two ways: entering keywords in a single search or searching for each term individually and then combining the results. In both strategies, the combination is performed using **Boolean operators**—these are *AND*, *OR* and *NOT*. Each works in a different way. Using *AND* will return results that contain *all* of the included terms. This is used to combine the major concepts—for instance, *handwashing AND barriers AND nurses*. Using *OR* will return results that include at least one of the terms; it is mainly used to combine synonyms—in this example, *barriers OR obstacles*. The Boolean operator *NOT* will return results that include the first term but exclude the second; it can be useful to exclude a particular subset of articles that are not wanted. For example, Yasmin may want to exclude articles relating to surgical scrubbing; in this case, she might use the search *handwashing NOT surgical scrubbing*.

Another issue to be aware of is that certain words can be spelt in different ways, while others can be used in different grammatical forms. Keyword searching will identify only articles that use the same spelling or form that you have used. Spelling usually varies by a single letter—for instance, *oesophagus* in the United Kingdom and Australia is spelt *esophagus* in the United States, and *paediatric* as *pediatric*. Both spellings can be included in a search (for example, *oesophagus OR esophagus*). However, most databases have a wildcard option that allows the searcher to insert a character in the place of a letter that may or may not be present; the specific character varies between databases but in MEDLINE is a question mark. The keyword in this example would be entered as *?esophagus*.

Variations can also occur in forms of words: in Yasmin's example, the concept of *nurses* may have been expressed by different authors as *nurse* or *nursing*. Rather than including every variation on the term in her search, Yasmin can use a truncator symbol to do this for her: the terms are reduced to their common letters—in this case, *nurs*— and the truncator symbol is placed after them. In MEDLINE, the truncator symbol is an asterisk. In this example, the keyword will be entered as *nurs**. Note that truncation can also return unwanted results. For example, *nurs* is also the beginning of the word *nursery*. Including this term might find articles relating to childcare centres or kindergartens. Yasmin could exclude these by using the Boolean operator *NOT*: *nurs* NOT nursery*.

Activity 2.1   Searching a database

1 On your institution's library website, go to a database of your choice.
2 Read the information provided about the database to determine what the wild-card and truncator characters are in that database.
3 Using the keywords identified in the text above, carry out a search to find articles relating to barriers to nurses washing their hands.

Question for consideration

- Which parts of the search did you find difficult? Review these areas with your lecturer or a colleague.

As we have seen, when using keywords to perform a search, it is important to identify all the synonyms that may have been used in the literature. The drawback to this method is that if you miss some synonyms, you will not find literature that you may need. A way around this is to locate your search term within an established thesaurus of terms, or subject headings. These differ somewhat between databases. One thesaurus that is used by several databases, including MEDLINE, was developed and maintained by the US National Library of Medicine and is called Medical Subject Headings (MeSH). Mapping, or linking, terms to subject headings ensures that all related terms are searched for.

In MEDLINE, Yasmin types *handwashing* into the search bar and clicks on the box 'Map term to Subject Heading'. This takes Yasmin to a screen indicating that her term mapped to the MeSH term *hand disinfection*. At this point, she has a number of options. We will concentrate on two: a link labelled 'Continue' and a link from the MeSH term itself.

When Yasmin clicks on the box labelled 'Continue', she can see all the subheadings that have been used to index articles under this subject heading. If one or more of these were relevant to her topic, she could narrow her search at this point by ticking the relevant boxes. In this case, however, none is appropriate to her chosen topic, so she returns to the previous screen. By clicking on the subject heading itself she can see what is called the *tree*—the more specific and more general terms associated with the term. This tells her that the term above it—the more general term—in the tree is *hand hygiene*. She can also see how many articles are associated with each term. For each term, she can click on the information icon to see the *Scope* note—the definition of each term, how it has been indexed previously, related terms and all the terms that are included under this heading:

MeSH heading: **hand disinfection**

Scope: The act of cleansing the hands with water or other liquid, with or without the inclusion of soap or other detergent, for the purpose of destroying infectious microorganisms. Used for:

- disinfection, hand
- hand disinfection
- hand sanitization
- hand washing
- hand washings
- sanitization, hand
- scrubbing, surgical
- surgical scrubbing
- washing, hand
- washings, hand

MeSH heading: **hand hygiene**
  Scope: Practices involved in preventing the transmission of diseases by hand. Used for:

- hand hygiene
- hygiene, hand (Ovid Technologies, 2023)

Yasmin can now decide which of the terms she wants to use, or she can select both. To include both terms in her search, she will need to combine them using the Boolean operator *OR*. She also has the option of ticking boxes either to *explode* the search (to include the term and any more specific terms) or to *focus* it (limit the search to articles in which the term is the major focus). Yasmin elects to choose both *hand hygiene* and *hand disinfection* and to tick the 'Focus' boxes for each. This operation elicits more than 5,000 articles—almost twice as many as were discovered by searching for the keyword *handwashing*.

MeSH headings are usually only useful for the main concept in a search, but it is worth trying the other terms to see if there is a suitable heading. *Barriers*, for instance, maps to a range of headings that have nothing to do with Yasmin's topic. *Nurses* is a MeSH term but retrieves only 5% of the articles identified by the keyword search for *nurs**. Unless the final search result elicits too many articles to reasonably examine, it is usually best to use a search strategy that will give the most results.

Once Yasmin has combined the searches on the individual terms (using the operator *AND*), she can narrow the results even further by using the 'Limits' function. One limit used frequently is the publication year. Whether to use this and which years to choose depend on the purpose of the search. If you want to know the most recent findings on a topic, restricting the search to the last five or ten years is a useful rule of thumb. However, if you want to know whether *any* research on your topic has been undertaken, you may need to go back further. For example, the link between lack of hand hygiene by healthcare workers and infections among patients is well established, and you would be unlikely to find recent research on that exact topic. (You might, however, find research on the comparative effectiveness of different types of hand hygiene.) There may be a specific time point at which practices changed (for example, the introduction of new laws or guidelines) that would influence the literature on a topic, so it would make sense to search for articles published only after that date. In Yasmin's case, she will need to retrieve articles only from the last five years, to comply with her assignment instructions. Another available option is to limit the search to articles written in English; this can be useful if the searcher can read no other languages and does not have translation resources. If relevant to the topic, other limits that can be applied include people's ages, types of articles and subsets of journals or subjects. Another option is 'Full text available'; this restricts the search to those articles to which the database has a full text link. This is not the same as a library's full text availability, which is any journal to which the institution subscribes. It is best, therefore, *not* to use this limit in your search, even when finding information for assignments.

All the concepts we have discussed in this section are illustrated in Table 2.2, which shows the results of the various searches and the effects of applying limits. As we saw above, applying the full text limit excludes a significant number of articles that Yasmin could use in her assignment. The best search strategy in this case has given her 21 articles to examine further. Note that no search strategy, however carefully designed, is foolproof, and there will likely be a number of retrieved citations that are not relevant to your specific topic. There is no way to avoid the final step, which is to read the titles and abstracts of the retrieved articles, to determine which ones will meet your needs.

Table 2.2 Results of searches conducted in MEDLINE concerning barriers to handwashing in nurses

Search number	Searches	Results
1	"barriers to nurses washing their hands"	0
2	hand hygiene OR hand disinfection [MeSH terms, focused]	5177
3	handwashing [keyword]	2981
4	barriers OR obstacles [keyword]	232143
5	nurs* [keyword, truncated]	810579
6	nurses [MeSH term]	45829
7	2 AND 4 AND 5	59
8	limit 7 to English language and year=2018-current	21
9	limit 8 to full text	5

Source: Adapted from Ovid Technologies (2023).

Activity 2.2   Constructing a strategy to search the literature

Choose any topic of interest to you and consider how you will go about finding research evidence on that topic.

Questions for consideration

- Which databases are likely to include articles relevant to your topic?
- Are there any MeSH terms relevant to your topic?
- What keywords could you use? Could these be spelt in different ways? What synonyms might have been used for these terms?
- How will you combine these terms in a search?

Research Example 2.1   Do nurses source research evidence?

Nurses and midwives have a professional responsibility to use evidence in their practice, but to do so they must be able to locate relevant and good-quality evidence. Fossum et al. (2022) conducted an integrative review of 52 studies from 16 countries, to describe the information sources that nurses use to inform their practice. Peers, reference material and computers were the most commonly cited sources across all study methods. Nursing journals were the 4th ranked source in quantitative studies, and 10th ranked in qualitative studies. How computers are used for finding information—the types of resources and the search methods, and thus the quality of the information sourced—could not be determined. The authors concluded that nurses need education and support to enable them to access good-quality evidence to inform their practice.

Fossum, M., Opsal, A. & Ehrenberg, A., 2022, 'Nurses' sources of information to inform clinical practice: An integrative review to guide evidence-based practice', *Worldviews on Evidence-Based Nursing*, vol. 19, pp. 372–379. doi: 10.1111/wvn.12569.

Questions for consideration

- What do you consider to be the implications of these findings for nursing practice?
- What strategies could be put in place to increase nurses' skills in finding and using research evidence?

How do I judge evidence?

In Chapter 1, we introduced you to the concept of hierarchies of evidence. This concept is underpinned by the fact that research evidence can be generated using several approaches, or study designs, and these do not all provide the same weight of evidence. Put simply, some designs are better suited to answering certain types of questions than others. Hierarchies of evidence were first developed to consider questions of effectiveness of various practices in producing a particular outcome, and they enable us to judge how confident we can be that the results of a study are 'real', or valid. For example, in the previous chapter, we looked at a systematic review that asked whether interventions to improve nurses' compliance with hand hygiene compliance were effective (Doronina et al., 2017). In this example, the evidence hierarchy helps us to judge whether the reported increase in compliance was due to the interventions or to some other factor. Some study designs include elements that enable us to have more confidence in the findings; hence, some designs are ranked higher than others. We will discuss these designs, and their various elements, in detail in subsequent chapters. Several organisations have published evidence hierarchies; the majority of these, such as the one illustrated in Chapter 1, relate to studies of effectiveness of interventions. In these hierarchies the various types of studies (described in Chapter 4) are assigned to a numbered level, which makes it easy to describe the quality of evidence when preparing literature reviews (see Chapter 9) and clinical practice guidelines (see Chapter 8).

Evidence-based health care is not simply about practice effectiveness; however, healthcare professionals have other questions, and research approaches designed to answer those questions can also provide evidence for practice. Other evidence hierarchies address those approaches. In nursing and midwifery, we are often interested in people's experiences, perceptions or behaviours, using qualitative approaches (see Chapter 5) to answer these questions. These concerns are categorised by the Joanna Briggs Institute (2014) as questions of 'meaningfulness'. The JBI has produced an evidence hierarchy for these types of studies:

a   Qualitative or mixed methods systematic review
b   Qualitative or mixed methods synthesis
c   Single qualitative study
d   Systematic review of expert opinion
e   Expert opinion (Joanna Briggs Institute, 2014)

Activity 2.3   Levels of evidence

1 Using the search strategy you developed in Activity 2.2, choose any two of the retrieved research reports.
2 Examine how the authors describe the type of research (which may be called *design, method* or *methodology* depending on the approach and the journal's style).
3 Try to identify the level of evidence that would be ascribed to the research.

Questions for consideration

• Was it easy or difficult to identify the level of evidence? Why was that?
• If it was difficult, what additional information could the authors have provided to assist in making this identification?

The level of evidence tells us about the quality of the available evidence—how credible it is. However, when deciding whether or not to incorporate specific evidence into our practice, a number of other factors have to be taken into consideration. This topic is explored in more detail in Chapter 8, in the discussion of clinical practice guidelines. Briefly, recommendations for the use of evidence in practice are graded as strong or weak and take into account the feasibility and appropriateness of a practice, as well as its meaningfulness and effectiveness (Joanna Briggs Institute, 2014).

Chapter summary

Locating high-quality evidence is a vital first step in evidence-based practice. This chapter has examined potential sources of research evidence and considered the relative credibility of each. Strategies to locate research evidence have been described. The need to consider the quality and strength of evidence when making decisions about its use in practice has been considered.

Chapter review questions

• What are the best sources for nursing and midwifery research evidence?
• Why are some sources considered better than others?
• What steps would you undertake in finding research evidence on a specific topic?
• What are Boolean operators? What functions do they perform?
• What do hierarchies of evidence tell us?

Questions for discussion

• Why is it important for nurses and midwives to undertake effective literature searches?
• Why is it important to understand evidence quality? How does this impact on clinical practice?

Questions for personal reflection

- What have you learnt about finding and evaluating research evidence while working through this chapter?
- How can you incorporate this knowledge into your practice?

Useful web resources

Centre for Evidence-based Medicine <https://www.cebm.ox.ac.uk/>.
Joanna Briggs Institute <http://joannabriggs.org>.
National Health and Medical Research Council on research <www.nhmrc.gov.au/research>.
US National Library of Medicine's Medical Subject Headings <www.nlm.nih.gov/mesh/>.

References and further reading

Aromataris, E. & Riitano, D., 2014, 'Constructing a search strategy and searching for evidence. A guide to the literature search for a systematic review', *American Journal of Nursing*, vol. 114, no. 5, pp. 49–56.

Briscoe, S., 2023, 'Errors to avoid when searching for studies for systematic reviews: A guide for nurse researchers', *International Journal of Older People Nursing*, vol. 18, no. 3, p. e12533. doi: 10.1111/opn.12533.

Considine, J., Shaban, R.Z., Fry, M. & Curtis, K., 2017, 'Evidence based emergency nursing: Designing a research question and searching the literature', *International Emergency Nursing*, vol. 32, pp. 78–82.

Doronina, O., Jones, D., Martello, M., Biron, A. & Lavoie-Tremblay, M., 2017, 'A systematic review on the effectiveness of interventions to improve hand hygiene compliance of nurses in the hospital setting', *Journal of Nursing Scholarship*, vol. 49, no. 2, pp. 143–152.

Eriksen, M.B. & Frandsen, T.F., 2018, 'The impact of patient, intervention, comparison, outcome (PICO) as a search strategy tool on literature search quality: A systematic review', *Journal of the Medical Library Association*, vol. 106, no. 4, pp. 420–431. doi: 10.5195/jmla.2018.345.

Fossum, M., Opsal, A. & Ehrenberg, A., 2022, 'Nurses' sources of information to inform clinical practice: An integrative review to guide evidence-based practice', *Worldviews on Evidence-Based Nursing*, vol. 19, pp. 372–379. doi: 10.1111/wvn.12569.

Joanna Briggs Institute, 2014, *Levels of Evidence*, <http://joannabriggs.org/jbi-approach.html#tabbed-nav=Levels-of-Evidence>.

Lawless, J. & Foster, M.J., 2020, 'Searching systematically and comprehensively', in C.E. Toronto & R. Remington (eds), *A Step-by-Step Guide to Conducting an Integrative Review*, Cham: Springer, pp. 21–44.

MEDLINE, Ovid Technologies Inc, 2023, Wolters Kluwer, details at https://www.wolterskluwer.com/en/solutions/ovid.

Section 2

How Can I Make Sense of Research Evidence?

Section 1 introduced the reader to evidence-based practice in nursing and midwifery along with the need for nurses and midwives to understand research in order to inform their practice. Trying to understand research papers can be daunting at first. They often use language and concepts that are new and appear complex. This section is focused on breaking down some of that complexity and providing the reader with a base on which to build research knowledge.

Chapter 3 introduces the research process. In doing so, it steps through each of the stages in conducting a research study, as well as some of the considerations needed. It introduces the concepts of quantitative and qualitative research, which are then built upon further in Chapters 4 and 5, employing a focus on person-centred care to illustrate their characteristics.

Chapter 4 introduces quantitative approaches to research, involving numerical, or statistical, analysis. The chapter presents basic statistical concepts commonly employed in nursing and midwifery research.

Chapter 5 introduces qualitative approaches to research, highlighting that these are particularly common in nursing and midwifery. It also discusses common approaches to data collection and data analysis, as well as ensuring research quality.

DOI: 10.4324/9781003414476-4

3 Understanding how research is done

Learning objectives

After working through this chapter, you should be able to:

- Describe the steps in the research process
- Outline the key differences between qualitative and quantitative approaches
- Define a *population* and a *sample*
- Identify potential sources of research data
- Outline formal and informal processes for gaining approval to undertake research
- Outline strategies for disseminating research findings
- Identify challenges that nurses and midwives might experience in collecting research data.

Key terms and concepts

Analysis, approval, data collection, population, qualitative, quantitative, research process, research proposal, research question, sample.

Case study overview

A large hospital has a strong philosophy that health care should be person-centred. At a meeting of senior nurses, there is a discussion around whether and how this translates into nursing practice. Nurse unit managers consider their own wards and departments and identify a number of issues and concerns. Some are uncertain about the extent to which person-centred care is being delivered and think this needs to be determined before proceeding with any further work. Others are certain that there are deficiencies in the delivery of person-centred care in their departments. Some of these think they should examine the reasons behind this, and others would like to look at ways of improving person-centred care.

Chapter introduction

Whether nurses and midwives want to undertake their own research or use existing evidence in their practice, an understanding of how research is actually carried out is fundamental to effective care. Every research study consists of a number of steps, which are known collectively as the research process. (This was described briefly in Chapter 1.)

DOI: 10.4324/9781003414476-5

The steps may not always be followed in exactly the same order, and the process may or may not be linear—sometimes steps can be revisited several times—but in general terms, the process is universal. This chapter describes in more detail the steps involved in planning and undertaking research. It introduces several concepts that will be explored in more depth in subsequent chapters.

Getting started: where do research questions come from?

Ideas for research can come from anywhere, but essentially they arise from a questioning attitude or from taking a critical approach to what we do. Ideally, we would constantly be asking questions about our practice—Why do we do something this way? Could we do it better?—but in the bustle of everyday life, it is very easy to just accept things the way they are. Questioning can be facilitated in a number of ways: reading journal articles, going to conferences, talking to colleagues (particularly those in other departments or hospitals), listening to those for whom we care or simply reflecting regularly on our work.

   Research begins with a broad topic of interest. In this chapter's case study, person-centred care is the broad topic. From this, researchers identify an issue or problem that they wish to address. In the case study, these problems are:

• uncertainty about whether person-centred care is delivered,
• wanting to understand why person-centred care is not being delivered consistently and
• wanting to improve the delivery of person-centred care.

Practice does not have to be perceived as a problem in order for us to investigate it. Rather than asking why something does not work, we might ask why it does! For instance, staff in some wards might decide that they practise person-centred care very well indeed; they and other staff would be interested in what enabled staff in that ward to practise person-centred care when staff in other wards did not. In practical terms, though, it is usually much harder to question something that is working well than something that has obvious problems.

   The issues or problems listed above are still quite broad and are not specific enough to guide a research study. They need to be refined further to generate focused questions that can be answered through research. Within any broad topic, and often within issues or problems, there are several research questions that can be asked. Some examples of possible research questions arising from the issues listed above are as follows:

• To what extent is person-centred care being practised throughout the hospital?
• What are the factors that facilitate or prevent the practice of person-centred care?
• What are nurses' perceptions and understandings of person-centred care?
• What are patients' perspectives of the practice of person-centred care?
• Can a nursing education program improve the practice of person-centred care?

When reading research reports, you will probably find that questions such as the ones listed above are not actually included. More commonly, the research aim is expressed as a statement. However, it is important to realise that the aim of any research study is to find the answer to a question, whether expressed as such or not—it is, effectively, to generate new knowledge. The aim of a study is not to change practice or improve patient

Research Example 3.1   Why do a literature review?

There is a great deal of literature, in nursing and other health professions, on the topic of person-centred care, and a number of different types of literature review have been undertaken.

Byrne et al. (2020) undertook an integrative review of the literature to develop an understanding of how the concept is applied in practice. Their review addressed two questions:

- Is there a generally accepted definition of person-centred care (PCC) that is used by nurses?
- How do nurses operationalise PCC in practice?

The review included 17 articles published between 1998 and 2018. The authors found that no single definition of PCC was used across studies, although there were core common themes. There were differences across clinical specialities, with some elements of PCC assuming more importance than others depending on the clinical context. Furthermore, they found a lack of alignment between the theoretical concept of PCC and how it was actually practised.

Byrne, A.L., Baldwin, A. & Harvey, C., 2020, 'Whose centre is it anyway? Defining person-centred care in nursing: An integrative review', *PLoS ONE [Electronic Resource]*, vol. *15*, no. *3*, p. e0229923. doi: 10.1371/journal.pone.0229923.

In another type of review, Rossiter et al. undertook an umbrella review of systematic reviews to assess the impact of person-centred care interventions on patient safety, across all healthcare settings. In the 16 reviews included, the majority of study participants were older adults, with only one review focussing exclusively on children, and none in maternity care. They found a wide range of interventions had been tested, with various aspects of patient safety as outcomes. Results of the studies were mixed, but overall indicated that person-centred approaches to care could contribute to patient safety. The authors concluded that there was scope for further high-quality research in this area and noted that as person-centred care is a complex topic, evaluating its impact requires a range of methodological approaches.

Rossiter, C., Levett-Jones, T. & Pich, J., 2020, 'The impact of person-centred care on patient safety: An umbrella review of systematic reviews', *International Journal of Nursing Studies*, vol. *109*, p. 103658. doi: 10.1016/j.ijnurstu.2020.103658.

Questions for consideration

- How might these papers assist staff in our case study to refine their research question?
- What types of research questions or problems might each study assist in developing?
- How else might they be useful to someone planning research on this topic?

outcomes; this is the significance of a study, or what you hope to achieve with the findings. It is helpful, therefore, to express an aim in the form of a question rather than a statement, because it focuses on the desired answer.

Moving from a problem to a research question requires some understanding of the topic and of what research has already been undertaken. Therefore, a literature review is usually undertaken at this stage. One reason for doing this is to identify gaps in current knowledge. It may be that there is already sufficient research evidence on a particular topic and the identified problem can best be addressed by implementing this evidence. It is unethical to conduct research unnecessarily—a topic we will explore further in Chapter 7. If more research is found to be justified, the literature review can be helpful in planning the study. Replicating another researcher's design makes it easier to compare findings across studies. The literature review can further help to refine the question by identifying existing measurement tools (to measure person-centred care, in this example) or interventions (like an education program) that have previously been tested.

Selecting an approach

There are two main broad approaches to undertaking research, known as **quantitative** and **qualitative**, which will be discussed in depth in the next two chapters. Here, we provide a brief overview, highlighting differences between the two approaches; these are summarised in Table 3.1.

It is important to understand that all research approaches are underpinned by a particular view of the world (known as a paradigm) that includes assumptions about the nature of reality, about what it means to be a person and about how knowledge can and should be generated. You will often see the word methodology used to encompass how these beliefs and assumptions shape the way research is undertaken (Johnston & Dowling, 2023; Ryan, 2018). The two research approaches are useful for answering different kinds of questions; therefore, the question will tend to determine which approach is chosen. However, the researcher's own philosophical beliefs will also influence the choice: they are more likely to be interested in asking questions that are best answered by the approach that aligns most closely with their beliefs.

Quantitative research

Quantitative research can be thought of as relating to numbers. It is primarily concerned with *measuring* concepts of interest and often with comparing the measurements to test theories. Questions about the effectiveness of practices—Do they have the effect we want to see? Are they better than other practices? If so, by how much?—are addressed using a

Table 3.1 Differences between quantitative and qualitative research approaches

Attribute	Quantitative	Qualitative
View	Objective	Subjective
Perspective	One truth or answer	Multiple truths
Focus	What, how much	How, why
Design	Usually fixed	Usually evolving
Data types	Numbers, information	Words, text, pictures
Data analysis	Statistical	Content, thematic

Activity 3.1   Questions suitable for quantitative and qualitative approaches

Read the list of possible research questions relating to the broad topic of person-centred care earlier in this chapter.

Questions for consideration
- Which questions would be best answered using a quantitative design? Why?
- Which would be appropriate for a qualitative design? Why?

---

quantitative approach. Quantitative methods are based on the assumptions that there is one *truth*, or answer, to the questions posed and that researchers (and all of the methods used) must remain objective in order to discover the truth. All elements of the research design are determined before commencing, with little opportunity for change once the research is under way. Data for quantitative studies are collected or expressed numerically and analysed using statistical methods.

Qualitative research

Qualitative research can be thought of as relating to words and behaviours, with findings 'telling a story' to answer the research question. It is concerned with how people experience, perceive or understand the concept of interest or with why they behave in certain ways (Johnston & Dowling, 2023). Qualitative approaches are based on the assumption that there are multiple *truths*—that people define their own reality, either as individuals or as part of a social group—and that no individual view is more or less true than another (Taylor & Francis, 2013). In other words, everything we research using these approaches is inherently subjective. Qualitative research designs often evolve as the research progresses: the number of participants, data sources and exact kinds of data may change as new information emerges.

Mixed methods research

A third research approach, mixed methods, usually involves combining quantitative and qualitative approaches. This approach is useful for answering the complex questions that often arise in clinical practice or for addressing a series of questions on the same topic to solve a practice problem (Cresswell & Plano-Clark, 2018). For example, researchers might use a qualitative approach first (for instance, to understand why person-centred care is not practised in a specific ward) and then a quantitative approach (to evaluate an intervention to improve practice). Researchers undertaking quantitative experimental studies (see Chapter 4) to see if new practices improve patient outcomes often include a qualitative component to understand patients' experiences of the new practice. Thus, mixed methods studies aim to produce more rounded findings that are better able to influence practice than either quantitative or qualitative approaches alone. A mixed methods approach is complex, requiring skills and knowledge beyond simply understanding each of the component approaches, and we will not be considering it in depth in this text.

Research Example 3.2   Using mixed methods to study person-centred midwifery care

Person-centred care in midwifery practice is widely acknowledged as being essential to ensure optimum outcomes for mothers and babies. However, most research on the topic has been undertaken in Western countries. Ogbuabor and Okoronkwo (2021) undertook a mixed methods study to understand how Nigerian midwives perceived person-centred care. The authors first surveyed midwives (quantitative component) to measure the extent to which they thought they provided person-centred maternity care (PCMC). They then conducted a number of focus group discussions (qualitative component) to gain deeper understanding of the midwives' experiences of providing PCMC. The qualitative data provided explanation and contextualisation of the quantitative findings, thus giving a more complete answer to the research question.

Ogbuabor, D.C. & Okoronkwo, I.L., 2021, 'Midwives' perspectives on person-centred maternity care in public hospitals in South-east Nigeria: A mixed-method study', *PLoS ONE [Electronic Resource]*, vol. 16, no 12, p. e0261147.

Questions for consideration

- Why was a mixed methods approach useful for this study?
- What might be the limitations of this study if the researchers had only chosen one method?
- This study relied on midwives' own reports of their practice to explore how well PCMC was practised. What are the advantages and disadvantages of this approach? How might a broader understanding of practice be achieved?

Activity 3.2   Differences between quantitative and qualitative research

1 Search for two research articles on a topic of interest to you, one quantitative and one qualitative.
2 Carefully read both articles, taking particular note of the research question or aim, the methods and the presentation of the findings.

Questions for consideration

- What differences do you see in the ways the studies are reported?
- Was the approach used in each of the papers appropriate? Why?
- Could the questions have been answered another way?
- What do you consider to be the strengths of each study?
- Which of the articles did you find easier to read? Why?
- Which of the studies did you find easier to relate to? Why?

Writing the research proposal

As part of the research planning process, researchers usually write a **proposal**, which is a blueprint for their intended study. A proposal can be written solely for the research team, to ensure everyone has the same understanding of what will be involved. Often, though, it is intended for external use: to gain approval by an ethics committee or an institution, or to obtain funding. The exact format varies somewhat, depending on the purpose, but generally describes how the researchers will complete each of the steps in the research process (see below).

A good research proposal sets the scene for the proposed study. It justifies the need for the study, by exploring what is already known on the topic and identifying a gap in current knowledge that the proposed research will fill. It has a clearly expressed aim and contains detailed but concise descriptions of all procedures. The importance, or significance, of the research, both to the wider community and to specific stakeholders, must be clear. Ethical considerations are usually discussed. Proposals intended for external scrutiny, such as by funding bodies, must convince their readers that the study can be conducted: the researchers have sufficient knowledge of their topic and expertise in research to undertake the study; there is sufficient time to complete the study (a detailed timeframe is usually included); and there are sufficient resources to complete the study, or the requested funding is appropriate (this requires submission of a detailed budget). Research proposals are examined in more detail in Chapter 11.

Seeking approval

Before the study can begin, researchers have to obtain approval from a number of sources. The first priority is ensuring all the proposed procedures are ethical. All research involving humans must be reviewed by one or more ethics committees. Approval is also required from the institution in which the research is to be undertaken—that is, where the research participants are located—and usually from the institution where the researchers are located, if this is different. For instance, university staff or students undertaking research in a hospital would need approval from both the university and the hospital. We will look in detail at what constitutes ethical research, and the work of ethics committees, in Chapter 7.

Permission to undertake the study might also be required from other people or institutions. The head of a department where the research will be undertaken will probably need to allow access to the department, to ensure that normal work is not disrupted by the research. This approval process often forms part of the ethical review. If participants are not within a specific institution but sought through other channels (such as professional organisations, support groups, social networks and so on), those bodies will need to approve the study. For some specific types of research, notification of various bodies is required. In Australia, for example, research involving drugs or devices that are either not registered in Australia or not approved for use in the way they will be used in the research must be reported to the Therapeutic Goods Administration, which will monitor the progress of the study. In most countries, randomised controlled trials (see Chapter 4) must be registered in a publicly accessible database before participants are enrolled (World Medical Association, 2013). This is partly to ensure that the study and therefore its findings are genuine and partly to assist people who might benefit from participating in a trial to find studies that could be suitable for them. The World Health Organization has a list of trial registries that it endorses (https://www.who.int/clinical-trials-registry-platform/network/primary-registries), as does the International Committee of Medical Journal Editors (https://www.icmje.org/about-icmje/faqs/clinical-trials-registration/). In the UK, trials are usually registered with ClinicalTrials.gov, an international registry. Australia and New Zealand jointly maintain their own Clinical Trials Registry, which can be accessed at www.anzctr.org.au.

Formal approval and notification processes are not researchers' only considerations. Informal processes can also come into play if key people in the research setting can influence how, or indeed whether, the research is undertaken. These people are known as *gatekeepers*, and their cooperation is crucial in successfully conducting research. Gatekeepers may have a role in providing access to potential participants, perhaps notifying a member of the research team of suitable candidates or passing information to people who might be participants. Sometimes, particularly in larger studies, staff may be asked to comply with study procedures; for instance, clinicians may need to carry out a specific nursing or midwifery practice in a specific way. A number of factors can influence gatekeepers' cooperation. Research that is seen as burdensome or difficult for clinicians or the department as a whole, particularly if it impacts on workload, is less likely to elicit cooperation. Similarly, staff are less likely to comply with procedures they perceive to be harmful or potentially harmful to patients (whether or not their perceptions are accurate) or if they see the research as unimportant. Even when they wish to cooperate, however, busy clinicians can forget about research in the press of daily work. The attitude of researchers can have a considerable influence on gatekeepers. Requesting assistance and rewarding compliance are more likely to produce a favourable response than complaints and recriminations.

Selecting participants

Before making decisions about who will take part in the research, we first need to identify the target population—the people who will be the focus of the research question. A population is defined as a group of people with common characteristics to whom we want the results of our research to apply. Usually, this means the people we can access. In any of the possible studies being undertaken in our case study, the population might be all nurses in the hospital. However, if we believe there are important differences between the practices of nurses in various departments, the population will be defined as nurses working in a department or ward where the study is taking place. If we want our population to be 'all nurses working in medical wards in public hospitals in Australia', we will need to include a number of such hospitals in the study to be able to apply our findings to this group.

Sometimes it is possible to study the whole population, particularly if it comprises a relatively small number of individuals. In the above example, for instance, it would (at least theoretically) be possible to involve all the nurses in one ward or one hospital in a study. In other cases, research designs have been developed that allow researchers to study very large populations, such as all women giving birth in Australia. More often, though, it is not practical to include the entire population, so researchers must choose a subset to take part in the research. The subset is called a **sample**, and the act of selecting it is known as sampling. There are several ways of selecting a study sample; these vary between qualitative and quantitative approaches and even within each approach. We will discuss these in detail in the following chapters.

Activity 3.3   Research considerations

A great deal of preparation goes into a research study. Summarise in a series of bullet points what you see to be the key considerations in planning a study.

The sampling method is not the only decision researchers have to make with respect to their participants. They must also decide where they will recruit people (that is, what the study setting will be) and how many participants they need (the sample size). How this decision is made depends mainly on the research design. Researchers need to establish what characteristics they want the participants to have and whether there are characteristics that they do not want. These requirements are called inclusion and exclusion criteria. They also have to decide on a recruitment strategy—how they will let potential participants know about the study and, in turn, how people will let the researchers know they want to take part. Sometimes, researchers approach potential participants directly, in person; this is the commonest method when conducting clinical research with patients, for instance. In some situations, it may not be possible or desirable for the researchers to approach individuals directly. They may instead advertise the study by means of flyers in the settings where they want to recruit, in newspapers, by email sent via a contact (for example, nurse unit managers may be asked to send an email to all their staff, or a professional organisation to its members) or on social media platforms, such as Facebook and Twitter. In all strategies, researchers must have plans for providing people with information about the study and obtaining their consent to take part (we will discuss this further in Chapter 7), and for how those who agree will either contact the researchers or provide their data.

Collecting data

The term data refers to any information collected to answer the research question. Data can be classified as inherently *quantitative* (that is, the information exists in a numerical format: a person's age, weight, body temperature and so on) or as *qualitative*, or non-numerical (a person's gender, hair colour, favourite food, opinion about a particular issue and so on). In practice, this distinction is only partially useful, however.

Data can be collected in almost any format and from almost anywhere. Common sources are:

- **Directly from people themselves** Data can be collected by measuring physical attributes, either immediately (height and weight, blood pressure, temperature etc.) or at a later time (for instance, collecting blood or urine to measure substances such as cholesterol or glucose). We can observe people in specific situations. We can ask questions of people, either in person or through another medium (such as a written or electronic survey).
- **Directly from the environment** We can measure attributes such as room temperature, noise levels, light levels and available space.

- **Existing data about individuals** This can be a very convenient way of obtaining data as it is usually less time consuming than sourcing it directly, although there are some disadvantages. Medical records are one such data source. Others are patient databases, which can exist at department, hospital/health service, state or even national level. Another example is patient registries, where details are recorded of patients with specific medical conditions (such as various cancers) or requiring specific types of care (such as intensive care admission).
- **Existing data about society or the context of a research project** This category can include policy documents, official records (such as incident reports in hospitals, birth and death records), published texts (books, newspapers, journal articles etc.) and other media (film, television etc.).

As well as deciding from where data will be collected, researchers must decide what data to collect. The data must enable the research question to be answered. This may sound simple (even obvious) but in reality can be complex and quite difficult. If the data are being collected by asking people questions, for instance, researchers must decide what questions to ask to get the information they want. Questions can be misunderstood by participants or just not specific enough to elicit the information. Even something as apparently straightforward as body temperature becomes more complicated when you consider that there are several sites on the body where temperature can be taken and several instruments that can be used to measure it, all of which might give slightly different readings. If we want to compare temperature across patients or across time periods, we need to take their temperature at the same site and using the same device every time. We also have to consider how many people will be collecting data. If more than one, it is important to ensure that everyone is collecting the data in the same way.

Other information must also be collected. Some demographic or clinical information will be needed to allow descriptions of the participants and enable the researchers (and those reading the research findings) to judge whether the sample is typical of the population or of a population in other settings. There is no standard list of items that should be included in demographic data. Rather, their relevance to the research question needs to be considered. Age might be important, for instance, when researching patients, as disease processes are likely to vary in different age groups. But if we are researching nurses' attitudes towards person-centred care, we might be less interested in their ages than in how long they have been practising as nurses. For research on patients, clinical data should be collected if it might influence the research outcome or help readers determine whether they should implement the findings. Finally, if the research involves the evaluation of an intervention, such as a new practice (see Chapter 4), the details of the intervention should be recorded to ensure that it is carried out in an identical way for all participants.

The format in which data will be collected also needs to be decided. A survey, for instance, could be paper based or electronic. If data collection is by observation, the situation might be filmed, or the observers may make notes about what they are seeing. Interviews with participants may be audio- or video-recorded, or the interviewer may write down the participants' responses. When physiological or clinical data are collected, they are usually recorded on a data collection form, which again may be in paper or electronic format.

Activity 3.4   Collecting research data

Data can be collected in many forms. Consider the possible challenges for nursing and midwifery researchers in collecting research data and suggest how these challenges might be managed.

Analysing data

Data analysis means making sense of the data that have been collected, in order to answer the research question. There are several ways in which this can be done, and they differ significantly between quantitative and qualitative approaches. In quantitative studies, statistical analysis is performed, and the results are presented in a numerical format. Often, tables and figures (such as graphs) are used to display the results. In qualitative studies, analysis is focused on finding patterns (themes or categories) in the data, and the findings are usually presented in narrative form. We will discuss specific methods of analysis in detail in the following two chapters.

Interpreting findings

This stage of the research process is undertaken to help consumers of research put the findings into context. You will see this stage in research reports under the heading 'Discussion'. The researchers consider how the findings of their particular study fit with what is already known on the topic: the findings may add further weight to a body of evidence, or they may challenge existing knowledge. Explanations should be suggested for new or unexpected findings; for example, the research may have been carried out in a different setting from that of previous studies or with people displaying different characteristics. The implications for practice (or policy or education, depending on the topic) should be discussed. Limitations of the study—factors that might restrict the application of the study's findings—should be identified. The researchers should also discuss what is still not known about the topic and suggest avenues for further research; there is a saying that good research asks more questions than it answers.

Communicating findings

The final stage of the research process is one that novice researchers often neglect to consider at the outset but is arguably the most important. If research findings are not communicated to others, the research might as well not have been done. It can be argued that failing to communicate findings is unethical, as people have taken part in research on the understanding that something useful will come of it. There are three groups of people to whom the findings should be communicated: participants, stakeholder groups and the wider scientific (and possibly lay) community. The communication of research findings is commonly referred to as **dissemination**. This is covered in detail in Chapter 10.

It is generally expected that people who have given up their time (at least) to take part in research should be given the opportunity to learn about its outcomes. Researchers are usually required, during preparation for the research, to formulate a plan for how they will communicate their findings. Normally, participants are told at the time of recruitment when the results are expected to be available and how to obtain them. If researchers have direct contact with the participants, they can offer to send them a summary of the findings. If there is no direct contact (in the case of an anonymous survey, for instance), the findings may be made available through a mutual contact.

Beyond the participants, a number of groups may have a specific interest in the study findings. Organisations that provide funding for research usually require a summary of the results. Approval bodies, such as ethics committees, often ask for a final report, which, while having a different focus, sometimes includes the study's findings. If research is undertaken in a specific organisation or environment, staff in the organisation will have a particular interest in the findings, as they are directly relevant to them. Staff will be specifically interested in the implications for their practice, especially if change is indicated.

For research to be relevant beyond the immediate setting, however, the findings have to be dispersed widely. This means they must be published in an academic journal, so that they can be read by both users of research and other researchers. This method of dissemination potentially reaches the biggest audience. Researchers can promote their work through a number of avenues to encourage others to read it, including social media platforms, blogs and membership of social networking sites like LinkedIn and Research-Gate. News media can also be used to draw attention to important research findings. Another useful way of disseminating findings to the scientific community is by presenting at conferences. This gives researchers direct contact with potential users of their research and with other researchers, allowing them to answer questions and discuss their work in detail. The disadvantage of this dissemination method is that a relatively small number of people are exposed to the research presented, compared with the potential audience of a journal article. Conference presentation should complement publication, not replace it. This topic is discussed in detail in Chapter 10.

Activity 3.5   Disseminating research findings through social media

Social media is a key mechanism by which scholars disseminate their research findings. There are a number of available social media platforms with which researchers should be familiar.

1 Go to one or more of the following websites:

- ResearchGate
- LinkedIn
- Academic.edu
- Google Scholar.

2 At each website, look for some researchers you may know in your discipline (for example, authors of articles you have read, your lecturers or people in clinical settings with whom you have worked). Note the types of information available on each site.

Chapter summary

Understanding how research is carried out is important for nurses and midwives, whether they want to do their own research or read research reports as the basis for decisions about their practice. In this chapter, we have explored the steps, or research process, involved in any research study. The first vital step is to generate an answerable research question located within what is already known on the topic through undertaking a literature review. There are two main approaches to research—quantitative and qualitative—and we have examined the differences between them. A third approach, mixed methods, was described briefly. The approach selected will guide subsequent steps, including selecting participants, collecting data and analysing data. Finally, it is vital to communicate research findings to others.

Chapter review questions

- What are the key differences between quantitative and qualitative approaches to research?
- What are the key decisions researchers must make in relation to how they carry out research?
- From what sources can data be collected?
- What strategies can researchers use to communicate their findings?

Questions for discussion

- How can nurses and midwives generate ideas for research?
- What are some of the challenges that nurses and midwives might face in undertaking research?
- What strategies could be used to promote research in nursing and midwifery practice?

Questions for personal reflection

- What have you learnt about doing research while working through this chapter?
- Based on your own philosophical beliefs, can you relate more to quantitative or to qualitative approaches?

Useful web resources

Australian and New Zealand Clinical Trials Registry <www.anzctr.org.au>.
International Committee of Medical Journal Editors. Clinical Trials Registration <https://www. icmje.org/about-icmje/faqs/clinical-trials-registration/>.
National Institutes of Health National Library of Medicine Online Database of Clinical Studies <https://www.clinicaltrials.gov/>.
World Health Organization Clinical Trials Registry Platform Network <https://www.who.int/ clinical-trials-registry-platform/network/primary-registries>.

References and further reading

Byrne, A.L., Baldwin, A. & Harvey, C., 2020, 'Whose centre is it anyway? Defining person-centred care in nursing: An integrative review', *PLoS ONE [Electronic Resource]*, vol. 15, no. 3, p. e0229923. doi: 10.1371/journal.pone.0229923.

Capili, B., 2020, 'How does research start?', *AJN, American Journal of Nursing*, vol. *120*, no. *10*, pp. 41–44.

Coyne, P., Kustra, E. & Woodruff, S., 2022, 'Let's talk about it: A narrative review of digital approaches for disseminating and communicating health research and innovation', *Journal of Public Health Management and Practice*, vol. *28*, no. *5*, pp. 541–549. doi: 10.1097/PHH.0000000000001518.

Cresswell, J.W. & Plano-Clark, V.L., 2018, *Designing and Conducting Mixed-Methods Research*, 3rd edn, Thousand Oaks, CA: Sage.

Fawcett, B. & Pockett, R., 2015, *Turning Ideas into Research: Theory, Design and Practice*, London: Sage.

Johnston, B. & Dowling, M., 2023, 'Qualitative research and cancer nursing: A guide for novice researchers', *Seminars in Oncology Nursing*, vol. *39*, no. *2*. doi: 10.1016/j.soncn.2023.151397.

Keeler, C. & Curtis, A.C., 2022, 'Secondary data in nursing research', *AJN, American Journal of Nursing*, vol. *122*, no. *4*, pp. 58–61.

Keeler, C. & Curtis, A.C., 2023, 'The architecture of a research study', *AJN, American Journal of Nursing*, vol. *123*, no. *5*, pp. 59–62.

Ogbuabor, D.C. & Okoronkwo, I.L., 2021, 'Midwives' perspectives on person-centred maternity care in public hospitals in South-east Nigeria: A mixed-method study', *PLoS ONE [Electronic Resource]*, vol. *16*, no. *12*, p. e0261147.

Rossiter, C., Levett-Jones, T., & Pich, J., 2020, 'The impact of person-centred care on patient safety: An umbrella review of systematic reviews', *International Journal of Nursing Studies*, vol. *109*, p. 103658. doi: 10.1016/j.ijnurstu.2020.103658.

Ryan, G., 2018, 'Introduction to positivism, interpretivism and critical theory', *Nurse Researcher*, vol. *25*, no. *4*, pp. 14–20.

Taylor, B. & Francis, K., 2013, *Qualitative Research in the Health Sciences: Methodologies, Methods and Processes*, Abingdon: Routledge.

World Medical Association, 2013, *Declaration of Helsinki: Ethical Principles for Medical Research Involving Human Subjects*, <www.wma.net/policies-post/wma-declaration-of-helsinki-ethical-principles-for-medical-research-involving-human-subjects/>.

4 Understanding quantitative research approaches

DOI: 10.4324/9781003414476-6

Learning objectives

After working through this chapter, you should be able to:

- Define the term quantitative research
- Describe the benefits of quantitative research for nursing and midwifery practice
- Outline the characteristics of experimental and non-experimental research designs
- Outline approaches to sampling in quantitative research
- Outline the key concepts of descriptive and inferential data analysis
- Describe approaches to ensuring validity and reliability in quantitative research

Key terms and concepts

Bias, case-control study, central tendency, cohort study, confidence intervals, confounder, cross-sectional study, data analysis, deductive, descriptive design, descriptive statistics, dispersion, experimental design, hypothesis, inferential statistics, intervention, measurement scales, non-experimental design, normal distribution, probability, quantitative, quasi-experiment, randomised controlled trial (RCT), reliability, sampling, skewed distribution, survey, validity, variable.

Case study overview

Stephanie and Marek are nurse unit managers in different wards in the hospital mentioned in the previous chapter. As discussed, the hospital has a strong commitment to person-centred care. Stephanie is not sure of the extent to which person-centred care is practised in her ward and thinks it would be a good idea to find out, as a baseline for further action. Marek, on the other hand, is sure that the nursing care provided in his ward is not as person-centred as it could be; he wants to investigate whether a nurse education program will improve the care. Both these concerns are appropriately addressed using quantitative approaches.

Chapter introduction

In the previous chapter, we introduced the concept of quantitative research as one of the basic approaches to undertaking research and generating new knowledge, concerned with measuring concepts of interest, testing theories and ultimately predicting outcomes. In this chapter, we will explore this approach in greater detail. We will examine the various ways of undertaking quantitative research—called designs—and the kinds of questions they are used to answer. We will also look more closely at how steps in the research process—selecting participants and collecting and analysing data—are undertaken in quantitative approaches.

What is quantitative research?

As we saw in the previous chapter, quantitative research is concerned with numbers—measuring, identifying relationships, explaining and ultimately predicting phenomena through the testing of theories. This is known as a deductive approach. Quantitative research methods originated in the so-called hard sciences, such as physics and chemistry, and have been adapted for use in researching people. The beliefs and values of those sciences dominate the way we do this sort of research. Quantitative researchers are concerned with 'facts', assuming there is only one reality, or 'truth'. In order to discover the 'true' answer, all external influences, including the presence of the researcher, must be minimised; thus, the researcher maintains an objective approach. Often, researchers will distance themselves as much as possible from the research process in order to achieve this. The people they research are often called 'subjects', which emphasises this objectivity, although many researchers argue against this terminology. For quite a long time, quantitative research was the only approach accepted in nursing and midwifery (Beyea & Slattery, 2013). While this view has changed, the approach is still highly relevant for answering many of the questions of concern to nursing and midwifery practice.

Quantitative designs

The aims of quantitative research can be to describe or explore something of interest, to examine associations between variables or to identify cause-and-effect relationships. In health care, cause-and-effect relationships that we are interested in include causes of disease and the effectiveness of our practices in achieving the aims of the care we provide, which might be prevention or cure of disease, reduction of symptoms, prevention of adverse events, patient satisfaction and so on. A number of research designs have been developed to answer questions relating to these aims. Broadly speaking, these designs can be categorised as either **experimental** or **non-experimental**. Non-experimental designs are often termed **observational** (which should not be confused with observation as a means of collecting data). Experimental designs are specifically focused on identifying cause-and-effect relationships. In this chapter's case study, Marek's question would be ideally answered using an experimental design, as he is interested in whether an education program results in, or causes, an improvement in person-centred care. Non-experimental designs can be used to simply describe phenomena of interest or to examine associations. Stephanie's question is suited to a non-experimental design, as she is interested in describing and measuring the current situation, without manipulating it in any way. Sometimes, cause-and-effect relationships can be inferred from non-experimental research findings, but we must be cautious in making such inferences. A comparison of quantitative research designs is provided in Table 4.1.

Experimental designs

The chief difference between experimental and non-experimental designs is the presence of an intervention. Here, intervention has a very precise definition. It is a procedure or practice that is administered or managed by the researchers. The details of the procedure are tightly managed and controlled to ensure that the subjects, or participants, experience it in exactly

Table 4.1 Comparison of quantitative designs

Designs	Intervention	Control group	Participant randomisation
Experimental			
RCT	Yes	Yes	Yes
1-group pre-post	Yes	No	N/A
2-group pre-post	Yes	Yes	No
2-group non-parallel	Yes	Yes	No
Non-experimental			
Cohort	No	Yes	No
Case-control	No	Yes	No
Cross-sectional, correlational	No	Occurs by chance, not actively sought	No
Descriptive	No	No	N/A

the same way. For example, researchers might be interested in whether vitamin D supplements can reduce the incidence of osteoporosis. In an experimental study, all participants would receive the same dose of the same preparation of the vitamin, the same number of doses per day, perhaps even taken at the same time of day, for the same duration. Hence, vitamin D supplementation would be the intervention. If the researchers simply studied the general public, who chose for themselves whether or not to take vitamin D, how much to take, when to take it and for how long—in other words, the researchers had no control over its ingestion—then it would not be an intervention, and the researchers would simply be observing the effects (hence, it would be an observational, or non-experimental, study).

Randomised controlled trial or true experiment

The best design for establishing cause-and-effect relationships is the **true experiment,** the classic version of which is the RCT. You may remember that in the evidence hierarchy in Chapters 1 and 2, this was ranked highest of the single study designs. This is because it provides the best assurance that the outcome of a study (in the above example, incidence of osteoporosis) is due to the intervention (vitamin D supplementation) and not to some other influencing factor, known as a confounder. There are several factors that could influence a person's susceptibility to osteoporosis: age, family history, calcium intake, diet and amount of exercise, for instance. There are three essential elements of an RCT:

1 **Intervention** An intervention, as already defined, which is administered to one group of participants (who may be called the **experimental, or study,** group).
2 **Control group** This is another recruited group, but it does not receive the intervention. It should be similar in every other way to the experimental group.
3 **Random allocation** The participants are allocated randomly to either the experimental or the control group. The aim of this process is to achieve even distribution of potential confounders (including ones we may not know about) between the two groups.

Importantly, the two groups participate in the study concurrently; therefore, the design is sometimes referred to as a **two-group parallel RCT**. The significance of this is that if any changes occur during the study period, it is highly likely that both groups will be affected in the same way. Randomisation can be made even more precise by a complex strategy called **stratified randomisation,** when known confounders are taken into account. You may come across this term in research reports, but it is not important to understand it at this stage.

An additional level of rigour in an RCT can be obtained by a process called **blinding,** or masking, which means that the group assignment is concealed, for the duration of the study, from the participants, the researchers, anyone who might be making decisions that could affect the outcome or all of these. In **single blinding,** the participants do not know to which group they have been allocated; this is usually achieved by giving a placebo (such as a sugar pill instead of vitamin D in the above example) to the control group. In **double blinding,** both the participants and the researchers remain unaware of the allocation. This minimises any risk of the researchers treating one group differently, either intentionally or otherwise, to influence the outcome. In clinical research, other people may be able to influence the outcome and should also be unaware of the group allocation. In the above example, for instance, the participants may have nutritionists advising them on their diet; the nutritionists may encourage one group to consume more calcium-containing foods than the other, which could interfere with the results. With some interventions, however, blinding is not possible. In our case study, for instance, Marek wants to test the effectiveness of a nurse education program, and it will be obvious to nurses whether or not they have participated in such a program.

RCTs do have some disadvantages. They usually require a lot of oversight by the researchers to ensure the procedures are strictly followed, which can be very costly. Other resources can be required too. The researchers need to have sufficient expertise themselves to be able to design and carry out the study or have expertise available through consultation (for example, statisticians). In some situations, it is not feasible to randomise participants. To return to our case study, if Marek were to conduct an RCT in his ward, he would randomly assign half the participating staff to receive the educational program, while the other half would be randomly assigned not to receive it. However, the two groups would be working side by side; if the members of the control group saw the experimental group practising differently, they might change their behaviour also, in spite of not having received the education. This is known as contamination of the two groups. If the outcome that Marek wants to measure involves the effect on patients, this would be even more problematic, as patients are likely to be cared for by nurses from both groups.

Another form of RCT is the **cluster randomised controlled trial.** This is designed to overcome the problems described in Marek's situation, where it would be very difficult to have the experimental and control groups in the same environment. In this type of study, the unit of randomisation is not the individual participant but a group of participants—in health care, wards or even entire hospitals are often used as groups. In Marek's case, if the hospital where he works is large enough and has several wards similar to his, he could carry out the study by randomising the wards to the experimental and control groups. If the number of available wards is too small, he could recruit similar wards to his from a number of hospitals, again randomly assigning the wards to the two groups. Cluster RCTs are much more difficult to conduct than other studies, usually needing a lot of resources, including financial, and often larger sample sizes than a simple RCT (Hemming et al., 2017). It is not usually an option for a small research team.

A relatively new variation on this is the **step-wedge cluster randomised controlled trial.** In this design, the groups—clusters—all begin the trial in the control condition and cross over to the intervention at specific time intervals—steps; by the end of the trial, all clusters are in the experimental arm. The randomisation determines the order in which the clusters cross over. The design enables comparison of the intervention and control both within and between clusters (Hooper & Eldridge, 2021). If Marek chose this option, he would take an initial set of measurements in each ward before introducing the education program. He would then introduce the program in each ward over a period of time, until eventually it was implemented in all wards. This design is said to closely mimic the way in which healthcare changes are introduced and evaluated and is particularly useful when it is difficult to remove an intervention—for example, the content of an education program cannot be unlearned. However, it may be prone to a higher risk of bias than conventional RCTs (Hemming & Taljaard, 2020).

Quasi-experimental designs

If a true experiment is not possible, then a **quasi-experimental design** is the preferred option. This means that either there is no control group, or there is a control group but the allocation is not done randomly. These designs are more prone to the effects of confounders and are therefore not considered as rigorous as RCTs.

Marek could carry out a quasi-experimental study just with the staff on his ward. He would first measure the level of person-centred care that is currently being delivered. He would then carry out the education program. Following this, he would measure person-centred care again to see if there was a difference from the first measurement. This is sometimes called a **pre-post test**. In this case, there is only one group, so there is no group to compare the results against. Any changes in nurses' practice could be due to the education program, but they could also be due to other factors; for example, nurses might have become interested in the topic when the first set of measurements was taken and obtained information themselves on which to base their practice. For this reason, this is considered the weakest of the quasi-experimental designs.

Marek could strengthen the design by including a control group. He could do this by measuring person-centred care on another, similar ward in the hospital where nurses did not participate in the education program. If nurses' practice in this ward did not change, while practice in his own ward, where nurses had participated in the program, did change, Marek could be more confident in attributing the change to the education program and not some confounding factor. However, because the nurses would not have been randomly allocated to either receive the education or not, he could not rule out the possibility that other factors had influenced the outcome. In this situation, the two groups would be studied at the same time, or in parallel, so there would be no confounding effect of different time periods.

Another quasi-experimental design—probably the commonest in clinical research—is known as the **two-group non-randomised non-parallel design**. In it, the outcome of interest is measured in one group, usually patients, exposed to current standard practice; this group functions as the control group. The intervention is then introduced as a change in practice, and the outcome is measured in another group, which is exposed to the new practice. In our case study, Marek could use this design if his outcome related to patients—for instance, patient satisfaction with nursing care. For this, he would measure satisfaction in a group of patients receiving care from nurses who had not been educated in person-centred care. He would then introduce the education program and measure satisfaction in another group of patients, receiving care from nurses who had been educated.

All the designs described in this section are subject to the influence of confounding factors, although the factors themselves vary between designs. Therefore, researchers—and users of research—need to be cautious in attributing any change in the outcome to the effect of the intervention. Hence, quasi-experimental designs are considered weaker than true experiments and are lower in the evidence hierarchy.

Non-experimental designs

Non-experimental designs are characterised by the lack of an intervention. They produce a lower level of evidence than experimental designs. However, sometimes the amount of evidence from non-experimental studies provides a compelling argument for a causative relationship. One example is the link between smoking and lung cancer. The evidence for this link was derived entirely from non-experimental designs, because it is impossible to test using experimental studies as people cannot be forced to smoke. In this case, the evidence was enhanced by laboratory research, which identified the mechanism by which smoking can lead to lung cancer. In the absence of this knowledge, we would still have to say that lung cancer is *associated with*, rather than *caused by*, smoking.

The simplest non-experimental designs are called **descriptive** or **exploratory**. As their names suggest, they are used when researchers simply want to describe and quantify a concept of interest. In our case study, Stephanie would use a descriptive design to measure person-centred care in her ward. She could do this in a number of ways, such as surveying nurses to ask about their practice or observing nurses to see how often they carried out certain practices; we will discuss this in more detail later in the chapter when we consider data collection.

Non-experimental designs can also be used to examine associations between the outcome of interest and other factors; when this is the intent they may be called **correlational designs**. For instance, Stephanie might be interested in whether nurses who have a postgraduate qualification practise person-centred care more than those who do not, or whether there are differences in practice between male and female nurses. She cannot control nurses' gender or their prior education, and therefore she cannot say that any difference she finds is caused by the factor; she can only say there is an association between the factor and the outcome. For this study, Stephanie would collect the data at a specific point in time and once only from each participant, making this a **cross-sectional design**. It is considered the weakest design in terms of establishing associations.

Two non-experimental correlational designs are **cohort** and **case-control designs**. Both are intended to examine associations and are considered more robust than cross-sectional studies, because researchers have more control over the selection of participants and the study conditions. Originally, the designs were developed in epidemiological research, to examine potential risk factors for diseases, and they have been adapted for use in clinical research. To describe these designs, we will return to the example given earlier in this chapter, that of a potential association between vitamin D supplementation and prevention of osteoporosis.

To conduct a cohort study, researchers would recruit a group of people (a cohort is, technically, a naturally occurring group—for example, people born in the same year or living in a certain area) who did not have osteoporosis and had not begun taking dietary supplements. The researchers would follow them over a period of time; they would ask them at regular intervals whether they were taking vitamin D, and they would record who developed osteoporosis. At the end of the study, they would calculate whether there was any difference in the incidence of osteoporosis between those who had taken the supplements and those who had not. A case-control study works in reverse. Researchers would find a group of people who had osteoporosis (cases) and ask them whether they had ever taken vitamin D supplements. They would then find another, similar group of people (controls) who did not have osteoporosis and ask them the same question. Again, they would then calculate whether there was a difference in the incidence of the disease. In both these designs, it would be difficult to attribute any reduction in osteoporosis directly to taking vitamin D—to say that taking vitamin D *caused* the reduction. Taking vitamin D could be part of a general lifestyle (healthy diet, exercise and so on) that would protect against osteoporosis.

Developing a research question

In quantitative approaches, the research question is usually precise and much narrower than in qualitative approaches. In Chapter 3, we looked at examples of broad questions that related to concerns around person-centred care. These questions would need further refinement for a quantitative study. The wording of the question should be congruent with the study design. For example, if Marek were proposing to undertake an RCT in a medical-surgical ward, his question could be *Do medical-surgical nurses who have undertaken a targeted education program practise person-centred care more frequently than nurses who have not?* If, on the other hand, he were to propose a one-group pre-post study, his question could be *Does the level of person-centred care delivered by medical-surgical nurses increase after undertaking a targeted education program?* As Stephanie is planning a descriptive study, her question could be broader—for example, *How frequently do nurses practise person-centred care in a medical ward?*

An important step in planning a quantitative study is to define the concepts in the research topic and how they will be addressed in the research; this is called operationalising the concepts and is usually necessary even with an apparently simple concept. If the concept were hypertension, for instance, we would need to define exactly what level of blood pressure constituted hypertension and which measurement (systolic, diastolic or mean) we were interested in. In our case study, person-centred care is a very broad concept,

---

Activity 4.1   Comparing quantitative research designs

- Search for two research reports on a topic of your choice that have used different quantitative designs.
- Read the papers carefully.

Questions for consideration

- How is the research question or aim expressed in each report?
- What are the differences between the papers in how they report the methods used?
- Are there any differences in the reporting of the findings?
- Is either of the designs easier to understand as reported in the article? Why?
- What are the implications of each article for your own practice?

and both Marek and Stephanie will have to decide how they are going to work with the concept in order to conduct research. They may decide to focus on an actual process of person-centred care, demonstrated through nurses' behaviours. In that case, they will need to work out what behaviours are person-centred and what are not, and whether they will focus on all or some of these. They may decide that nurses' attitudes are a good predictor of their practice and focus on measuring those. Alternatively, they may decide to focus on an outcome of person-centred care. This may be a general outcome, such as patient satisfaction with care, or something very specific, such as length of hospital stay or rates of infection. Thus, the research question could be refined even further once the operationalisation of the concepts had been completed.

As we have seen, the focus in quantitative research is on measuring concepts of interest. Any measured concept or characteristic that can vary in a study is called a **variable**. The actual measurements that can be obtained for a variable are termed its **values**. For example, the variable eye colour can have the values brown, blue, green and grey. The outcome of interest—in this case, person-centred care, however, we choose to operationalise it—is called the **dependent variable**. If we are interested in investigating the influence of a specific factor on the outcome, whether or not it is an intervention, it is called the **independent variable**. When the aim of a study is to examine relationships between variables, the research question is usually framed as a hypothesis, a statement about the assumed relationship, which the researcher can then test. The scientific method requires that this statement be framed in the negative: this is termed the **null hypothesis**. In Marek's experimental study, the null hypothesis could be *There will be no difference in the practice of person-centred care between nurses who have undertaken an education program and those who have not*. The study should be designed in such a way that the null hypothesis can be disproved (if in fact it is not correct). The **alternative hypothesis** is the opposite of the null hypothesis. The possibilities if the null hypothesis is wrong are twofold: person-centred care could be better if nurses have undertaken an education program, or it could be worse. The most scientific approach is to allow—and therefore test—for either of these possibilities. Therefore, the most appropriate alternative hypothesis would be *There is a difference in the practice of person-centred care by nurses who have and nurses who have not undertaken an education program*. This is called a **nondirectional hypothesis**, because it does not privilege one possibility over the other.

The next important step is to determine how the variables of interest will be measured. In quantitative research, we talk of measuring all variables, even non-numeric ones. In a broad sense, how variables are measured depends to a large extent on how we want to analyse the data to answer the research question. In Marek's study, he needs to be able to compare the level of person-centred care delivered by nurses at two points in time. To do this, he must reduce the dependent variable—person-centred care delivered by every nurse in the study—to a single numerical value. Therefore, he needs to find a tool that will enable him to do this. We will look at this further when discussing data collection. His independent variable—the education program—is simply measured as either having or not having been undertaken. The ways in which we can measure variables, whether numerical or not, are called **measurement scales**. These scales are:

• **Categorical or nominal** The values of variables represent a classification or group membership. Examples of variables include gender, hair colour, presence or absence of disease, and participation or non-participation in an education program. There is no logical order to differences between the values.

- **Ordinal** The values are ordered (ranked), but the differences cannot be quantified. Variables may be numerical (such as the order in which people finish a race or the ranking of people taking part in a contest) or non-numerical (such as army ranks).
- **Interval** Differences between values correspond to real, meaningful, consistent differences in the phenomenon being measured. In these variables, there is no **natural zero**; that is, a value of 0 does not represent an absence of the entity being measured. Examples include temperature in degrees Celsius and the year of an occurrence: 0 degrees Celsius does not indicate an absence of temperature, and the year 0 is not the point at which time commenced. What is more, this measurement is not subject to multiplication or division; 200 degrees Celsius is not twice as hot as 100 degrees Celsius, for instance.
- **Ratio** Variables that can be measured on the ratio scale are similar to interval variables in that differences between values are meaningful and consistent, but these variables do have a *natural zero*, indicating absence of the entity (for example, length, duration and weight), and can be multiplied and divided; 10 centimetres is twice as long as 5 centimetres, for instance.

Researchers need to understand these scales, as they largely dictate how data are analysed. The scales are considered as an ascending hierarchy, increasing in complexity from nominal to ratio. The more complex the scale, the more sophisticated the analysis that can be undertaken.

Research Example 4.1   Using a quasi-experimental design to improve person-centred care

Person-centred care of infants in Neonatal Intensive Care Units (NICUs) focuses on both the infant and their family, where it is known as Family-Centred Care (FCC) or Family Integrated Care. As a model of care it is known to improve health outcomes and wellbeing of infants and families and promote bonding of parents and babies; however, it may be challenging to implement. Toivonen et al. (2023) developed an education program for NICU staff to develop their ability to collaborate with parents. Parents and nurses evaluated the quality of FCC in the NICUs before and after the education program, using a tool developed for the study in collaboration with parents. Fathers rated FCC higher after the intervention than before, while mothers' scores were unchanged. Nurses also perceived that the quality of FCC improved after the intervention.

Toivonen, M., Lehtonen, L., Ahlqvist-Bjorkroth, S. & Axelin, A., 2023, 'Effects of the close collaboration with parents intervention on the quality of family-centered care in NICUs', *Advances in Neonatal Care*, vol. 23, no. 3, pp. 281–289.

Questions for consideration

- What features of this study design make it a quasi-experiment rather than a true experiment?
- Why might the researchers have opted to use this design rather than a true experimental design?
- How might the findings be applied to nursing practice?

**Research Example 4.2   Using a cross-sectional correlational design
to study woman-centred midwifery care**

Caseload midwifery care, in which pregnant women are cared for by a team of
midwives throughout their pregnancy, is believed to promote a woman-centred
approach to care. Women cared for by a small number of midwives, rather than a
large team, have fewer interventions and are more likely to be satisfied with their
care. Does this suggest that midwives working in smaller teams are more woman-
centred? Kuipers et al. set out to answer this question by surveying 553 pregnant
women receiving midwifery-led primary care in the Netherlands. They collected
data using a validated instrument called the Client Centred Care Questionnaire, to
measure interpersonal interactions between themselves and their midwives. They
found that, while all participants reported relatively high levels of woman-centred
care, women cared for in small practices (1–2 midwives) reported their care was
significantly more woman-centred than those cared for in mid-size (3–4 midwives)
or larger (≥5 midwives) practices.

Kuipers, Y.F., van Beeck, E., van den Berg, L. & Dijkhuizen, M., 2021, 'The comparison of
the interpersonal action component of woman-centred care reported by healthy pregnant
women in different sized practices in the Netherlands: A cross-sectional study', *Women &
Birth*, vol. 34, no. 4, pp. e376–e383.

Questions for consideration

- What do you consider to be the strengths and weaknesses of this study design?
- What features of the design make this study correlational rather than descriptive?
- What are the implications of the study for midwives?

Sampling and sample size

The aim of sampling in quantitative research is to select participants who will be representative of the population from which they are drawn; that is, the characteristics that are
important to the study should be the same in the sample and the population. The likelier
this representativeness is, the more confident researchers can be that the results of the
research can be applied (generalised) to the population. Sampling methods can be divided
into two categories: **probability** and **non-probability** methods. Probability sampling is
most likely to achieve a representative sample and is intended to give every member of the
population an equal chance of being selected. The strategies are outlined below.

Probability sampling

- **Simple random sampling** In this method, a random-number generator, usually in the
  form of computer software, is used to select the required number of participants from
  the population. There is no consideration of any specific characteristics.
- **Stratified random sampling** This method divides the population according to one or
  more characteristics, and a random sample is drawn from each. It is used to ensure

proportional representation of a characteristic; for instance, a population of nurses could be stratified into male and female. As males make up around 10% of the nursing workforce, a similar percentage could be selected to be in the sample.

- **Cluster random sampling** Here, the selection is of groups rather than of individuals; for example, a random selection of hospitals could be chosen for people within them to be involved in a study.
- **Systematic sampling** In this method, the participants are chosen not at random but according to a specific schedule; for example, if you were conducting research in women who had recently given birth, you might choose every third mother admitted to a postnatal ward.

Non-probability sampling

- **Convenience sampling** In this method, people are approached because they are readily accessible, and they self-select to take part. People responding to a survey usually constitute a convenience sample. People who feel particularly strongly about a topic or have extreme views may be more likely to take part than other members of the population and so are less likely to be representative.
- **Quota sampling** The intention with this method is to generate a sample with the same proportion of a characteristic as occurs in the population. Again, people self-select to take part, but they are accepted only until the quota is filled. To use the example of male and female nurses, male nurses who came forward would be accepted until the required number to form 10% of the sample size was reached.
- **Purposive sampling** This method involves hand-picking people with specific characteristics. It is rarely used in quantitative studies.

The number of participants needed for a quantitative study is usually determined before the study commences. In a descriptive study with a convenience sample, the sample size may be simply a pragmatic consideration—the number that can reasonably be expected to take part. The number required to provide a reasonable representation of the population can be calculated. In experimental studies, particularly RCTs, the sample size must be sufficient to enable detection of a true difference between the groups and is always calculated beforehand. This notion is rather complex but relates to the statistical concept of probability—that is, if we find there is a difference in the outcome between the experimental and control groups, we have to determine whether this occurred by chance or because of a real effect of the intervention. In analysing the data (which we will look at in more detail presently), we calculate, using a statistical test, the probability, or likelihood, of the difference occurring by chance. If the sample size is too small, the test result will suggest the finding occurred by chance. The likelihood that the test will correctly indicate a real effect of the intervention is called the power of the study.

Collecting data

Any of the sources of data described in the previous chapter can be used in quantitative studies. However, the format in which data are collected is very specific. As discussed above, data must be collected so that all variables can be measured in an appropriate way to answer the research question. For example, Stephanie could choose to collect data for her descriptive study by observing nurses in her ward. She would need to decide what specific behaviours by nurses constituted person-centred care or non-person-centred care and then record instances of these behaviours when they were observed. The nurses' activities could thus be quantified.

A specific type of data collection used in quantitative research is the survey, or questionnaire. In quantitative research, surveys usually consist mainly of closed-ended questions; that is, a finite list of answers is provided from which the participants must choose. One particular style of question that is often used in surveys is the **Likert scale** question. A Likert scale is a rating scale on which participants respond to a series of statements. Responses often range from 'Strongly disagree' to 'Strongly agree', or similar terms relevant to the question. Surveys can consist of related but independent questions designed to explore a particular situation. Surveys can also consist of questions that, when taken together, measure a specific entity, such as person-centred care, patient satisfaction or interprofessional collaboration. Developing a survey tool is a complex process with several issues to consider (Ruel, 2019). It is preferable to see if there is an existing tool suitable for the purpose of a planned survey. This not only saves time and effort; it enables results from studies using the same tool to be compared or data to be combined to enhance knowledge on the topic.

Analysing data

Analysis of quantitative data is almost always undertaken using computer software. Some analysis can be performed using a simple spreadsheet program, such as Microsoft Excel, while more complex operations require a dedicated statistical package. There are many of these on the market; one of the most commonly used, and supported by many institutions, is IBM SPSS. There are two levels of quantitative data analysis, known as descriptive and inferential. **Descriptive statistics** are used, as the name suggests, to describe data by summarising them. In a purely descriptive study, this would be the only level of

---

Activity 4.2   Designing a quantitative study

1 Using the concept of person-centred care, imagine you are planning a quantitative study with the focus on how nursing students understand the concept.
2 Choose one quantitative research design that you could use for the study.
3 Write a short, clear research question that could be answered using your chosen design.

Questions for consideration

- Where would you find the right participants?
- What sampling process would be appropriate for your study?
- How would you go about recruiting participants?
- What data would you need to collect to answer your question?
- How would you collect the data?

analysis performed. In other studies, it would be the first level of analysis. **Inferential statistics** are used to examine associations between variables and to draw inferences between the sample (in whom the measurements have been taken) and the wider population.

An important concept in data analysis is the normal distribution, in which data values, when presented graphically, form a symmetrical bell-shaped curve, with the majority clustered around the centre and the rest tapering out towards both ends (see Figure 4.1). Many large datasets will form this distribution. An asymmetrical distribution, with a longer tail at one end than at the other, is called a **skewed distribution** (see Figure 4.2). In a positively skewed distribution, the longer tail is to the right, while a negatively skewed distribution has a longer tail to the left. It is important to know whether data are normally distributed or skewed, as different analytic techniques are required for each.

Descriptive statistics

There are two types of measurements that are used to summarise data; they are referred to as **central tendency** and **dispersion**. Central tendency is the tendency of data to cluster

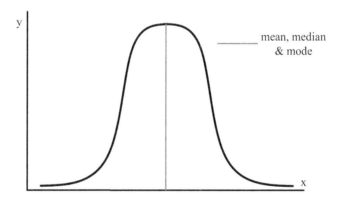

Figure 4.1 A normal distribution.

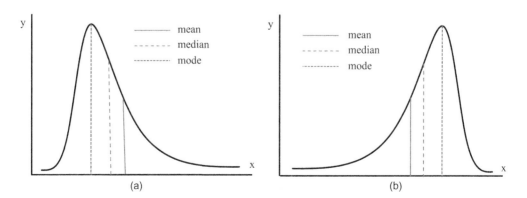

Figure 4.2 Skewed distributions: (a) positive skew, (b) negative skew.

around a point towards the middle of the range; this is illustrated in the bell shape of the normal distribution. Central tendency can be measured in the following ways:

- **Mean** The average of a set of numbers, obtained by summing all the values and dividing by the number of values in the dataset.
- **Median** The middle value when the values in a dataset are placed in numerical order; if there is an even number of values, the median is calculated by taking the average of the two middle numbers.
- **Mode** The most frequently occurring value in a dataset.

In a normal distribution, the mean, median and mode are all the same (see Figure 4.1). In a skewed distribution, the mean is pulled away from the median in the direction of the tail (see Figure 4.2) and is therefore less representative of the dataset.

Measures of dispersion tell us about the amount of variation in the data. The measures that can be used are:

- **Frequency** The count of the occurrences of values in a dataset expressed as a number, a percentage or a proportion.
- **Range** The difference between the highest and lowest values in a dataset.
- **Variance** In simple terms, the average of the differences between each individual value and the mean. To make the mathematical calculation possible, each of the values must be squared. This measure is rarely used in practice.
- **Standard deviation** The square root of the variance, in essence correcting for the squaring of values that occurred in calculating the variance. It is nearly always used in preference to the variance.
- **Percentile** The value at or below which lies a certain percentage of values in a distribution. For example, 10% of the distribution will lie below the 10th percentile. (Percentiles are used in clinical practice when tracking growth measures; infants' weight and head circumference and children's height, weight and body mass index are all tracked using percentile charts.) The 25th, 50th and 75th percentiles divide the distribution into quarters and are therefore called the 1st, 2nd and 3rd quartiles (and, of course, the 50th percentile, or 2nd quartile, is also the median, as described above).
- **Interquartile range** The difference between the 1st and 3rd quartiles; also known as IQR.

The measures of central tendency and dispersion are not interchangeable and should be used for specific scales of measurement; these are summarised in Table 4.2. Knowing how the measures are derived can be helpful in understanding their use, but it is no longer necessary to know how to calculate them: any computer program capable of data analysis will do this for you. It is more important to be able to interpret them, particularly measures of dispersion. The higher the dispersion, the more variability there is in the data, and hence the less the measure of central tendency represents the sample.

Inferential statistics

Inferential analysis examines associations between variables and provides information on whether results obtained from a study sample can be generalised to the population. The assumption underpinning this is that results may not be replicated exactly if the study were to be undertaken in another sample or if the findings were to be

Table 4.2 Descriptive statistics and when to use them

Measurement scale	Central tendency	Dispersion
Nominal (categorical)	Mode	Frequency
Ordinal		
Non-numerical variable	Mode	Frequency
Numerical variable	Median	Range, interquartile range
Interval, ratio		
Normal distribution	Mean	Variance, standard deviation
Skewed distribution	Median	Range, interquartile range

implemented into practice; that is, some variation would be expected. Data can be analysed using a wide variety of statistical tests using statistical software. Which test is used depends on a number of things, including what the researcher wants to know and what scale of measurement applies to the variables. Some of the simpler and more common tests, and the circumstances in which they are used, are listed in Research Tip 4.1. It is important that researchers understand what the various tests do and when they are used; the software cannot make this decision itself. There are two ways of assessing the statistical significance of associations between variables: through **probability** and **confidence intervals**. In older research reports, you are likely to see only probability mentioned, while in some recent reports, you may only see confidence intervals. However, both are often reported.

Probability is the likelihood of a result occurring by chance. It is represented by p or sometimes P, and it is expressed as a proportion of 1. Its potential range is from an infinitely small number to 1; that is, it can never be 0. To put it another way, we can never be absolutely certain that any finding is not due to chance alone rather than to a real effect of the independent variable. The smaller the number, however, the less likely it is that the finding is due to chance rather than to a real effect. Researchers choose in advance what limit they are prepared to place on this uncertainty; this is termed **statistical significance**, the upper limit of p at which they are prepared to claim their findings are due to a real difference in their data. By convention, the value of $p = 0.05$ is usually chosen; this means there is a 5 in 100, or 5%, likelihood of the results occurring by chance.

As an example, consider Marek's research in our case study. Let us suppose that when he measures nurses' person-centred care before the education program, he finds that the mean score across his sample is 50%; that is, they are practising person-centred care 50% of the time on average. The measure following the program is 65%—an increase of 15%. The statistical test results in a p-value of 0.03. This means there is a 3% probability of the result occurring by chance, which is a small value and below the conventional level of significance. Thus, Marek can reasonably attribute the change in nurses' scores to his education program and not to some random occurrence. On the other hand, if he obtained a p-value of 0.4, this would indicate a 40% probability that the result occurred by chance, and he could not assume that the difference was due to his program.

Confidence intervals provide a more precise way of judging whether findings can be generalised to a population. They indicate what the likely result would be in the population as a whole, or, to put it another way, they give an estimate of the true effect of the independent variable. Any confidence interval can be calculated, but it is conventional to use 95%; that is, we can be 95% confident that the true result lies between the calculated parameters. The wider the confidence interval, the more uncertainty there is in the truth of the findings.

Activity 4.3 Descriptive statistics and measurement scales

The table contains details of final marks and grades obtained by a class of 30 students.

Questions for consideration

- What is the appropriate measurement scale for each of the variables: status, gender, mark and grade?
- Calculate the mean, median and mode of the marks.
- From your answers to the above, do you infer that the distribution of marks is normal or skewed? Give reasons for your answer.

Student code	Status	Gender	Mark	Grade
1	International	M	90	HD
2	Domestic	M	67	C
3	International	F	55	P
4	Domestic	F	55	P
5	International	M	75	D
6	Domestic	F	88	HD
7	International	F	65	C
8	International	F	49	F
9	International	M	57	P
10	International	M	76	D
11	International	F	61	C
12	Domestic	M	82	HD
13	Domestic	F	75	D
14	Domestic	M	71	D
15	Domestic	F	65	C
16	Domestic	F	85	HD
17	Domestic	M	56	P
18	Domestic	M	40	F
19	Domestic	M	67	C
20	Domestic	F	54	P
21	International	F	36	F
22	International	M	65	C
23	International	M	87	HD
24	Domestic	F	52	P
25	Domestic	M	68	C
26	Domestic	F	53	P
27	Domestic	M	77	D
28	International	F	65	C
29	Domestic	M	42	F
30	International	F	72	D

Note: HD high distinction, D distinction, C credit, P pass, F fail.

Research Tip 4.1   Common statistical tests and their purposes

Chi square	Compares two categorical variables, each of which has two or more values
T-test	Compares a continuous (ratio or interval) variable between two groups
Analysis of variance	Compares a continuous (ratio or interval) variable between three or more groups; also known as ANOVA
Correlation	Compares two continuous variables when both are measured, not manipulated
Regression	Examines the effect of manipulating one continuous variable (the independent variable) on a continuous outcome variable (the dependent variable)

Let us return to the example above, in which Marek finds a 15% increase in person-centred care after his education program. Suppose he calculates the 95% confidence intervals to be 10 and 20: that would mean he can be 95% certain that the true effect of the program was to increase person-centred care somewhere between 10% and 20%. A reader could then judge whether it would be worth implementing the program or not.

Research rigour

In quantitative research, the main evaluation of research rigour is the extent to which it is free from bias. **Bias** has a very specific meaning in quantitative research: it is a systematic error in the way participants are selected, outcomes are measured or data are analysed that leads to results being inaccurate. All research designs are subject to bias to some degree, from various sources, but some are more susceptible than others.

Validity

The validity of research findings is their accuracy. In research designs that examine associations between variables, we distinguish between internal and external validity. Internal validity means that the outcome (dependent variable) is associated with or caused by the explanatory or independent variable rather than a confounding factor. Threats to internal validity include: attrition bias (participants dropping out or being lost to follow up); maturation bias (participants' characteristics or behaviour changing naturally over time); history bias (changes in the research setting during the course of a study); testing bias (changes to the outcome variable as a result of participants being tested); and instrumentation bias (changes to the instruments being used to measure the outcome, or how they are used). External validity refers to the extent to which findings can be generalised.

One aspect of research rigour is the accuracy with which variables are measured. When using any type of instrument to take measurements, we need to be certain that it has both validity and reliability. The validity of an instrument refers to whether it accurately measures what it is supposed to measure. For instance, a thermometer is a valid instrument of temperature measurement, but if we tried to use it to measure blood pressure, it would be invalid. Survey instruments—questionnaires—work in the same way. If we wanted to use a survey tool to measure an aspect of person-centred care, for example, we would need to make sure it was actually measuring that and not another concept.

Reliability

Reliability is the consistency with which an instrument measures the construct. The same result should be obtained if the measurements are taken repeatedly, so that changes in the measurement represent a real change in what is being measured. To return to the example of the thermometer, we would expect that if we used it to take someone's temperature several times in a short period, we would obtain the same result. We expect survey instruments to perform in a similar way. Research reports that have used a survey tool should report on both the validity and the reliability of the tool and how these were established.

Reporting findings

Reports of quantitative research share a very similar structure, whatever research design was used:

* **Background or introduction** This sets out what is already known about the topic and explains why the current research was undertaken.
* **Aim** This is usually phrased as a statement of purpose but may be phrased as a question; either way the intent of the research should be clear. A hypothesis should be included for experimental studies.

Research Example 4.3   Tools to measure person-centred care

When using an established tool in research, it is important to ensure that the tool is fit for the purpose for which it will be used—that it has validity (measures what we want it to measure) and reliability (measures the same concept consistently). This applies whether the tool is a survey instrument to be completed by participants, or an instrument used in direct observation, for instance to assess performance. Ekman et al. (2020) reviewed tools used to assess health professionals' competency in practising person-centred care. They found 16 tools used in 19 studies, which varied in their conceptualisation of person-centred care and the scope of what was measured; only two covered all dimensions. There was also variability in the reporting of reliability and validity evaluations. They concluded that all the identified tools had advantages and disadvantages.

Ekman, N., Taft, C., Moons, P., Makitalo, A., Bostrom, E. & Fors, A., 2020, 'A state-of-the-art review of direct observation tools for assessing competency in person-centred care', *International Journal of Nursing Studies*, vol. 109, p. 103634.

Questions for consideration

* How can articles such as this assist researchers?
* What are the implications of this study for nursing and midwifery practice?

Activity 4.4   Analysing a quantitative research paper

1 Locate a quantitative research paper on a topic of interest to you.
2 Carefully review the paper, examining the description of the data analysis in the methods section and the reported results.

Questions for consideration

• How were the data analysed?
• Are statistical methods clearly explained and tests named?
• Are p-values or confidence intervals, or both, reported?
• Are the results clear?
• What have the authors reported about validity and/or reliability?
• Have they identified potential sources of bias?
• Do the methods appear sufficiently rigorous to you?
• What do you consider to be the strengths and weaknesses of the report?

Research Tip 4.2   Reporting standards relevant to quantitative designs

CHEERS	Economic evaluations
CONSORT	RCTs; extensions for cluster and step-wedge trials
SQUIRE	Quality improvement studies
STARD; TRIPOD	Diagnostic and prognostic studies
STROBE	Observational studies

• **Methods** This section is particularly important, as this is what is mainly used to judge the rigour of the study. Moreover, the methods should be described in sufficient detail that another researcher could replicate the study. The section should include descriptions of the setting, the sample (including sample size and how it was determined), how participants were recruited, all study procedures, what data were collected and how, and how data were analysed.
• **Results** The findings are presented in this section, often in the form of tables or figures. There should be enough descriptive statistics for readers to judge the similarity between the study participants and the people to whom they would apply the findings. Results of statistical tests should be presented in a standard format without interpretation.
• **Discussion** This section interprets the findings and places them in context, discusses the implications of the results and identifies limitations of the study.

Reporting standards have been developed for a range of research designs (see Research Tip 4.2 for examples), and it is expected that all publications will follow them. This enables readers to judge whether the research has been undertaken rigorously and the degree of potential bias. The standards can be accessed through the EQUATOR (Enhancing the Quality and Transparency of Health Research) Network, at <www.equator-network.org>.

Chapter summary

Quantitative research is commonly used in nursing and midwifery research. It enables concepts to be quantified, either for purely descriptive purposes or to compare across different situations. It enables exploration of relationships between concepts (variables) and is particularly important in determining the effectiveness of practices and therapeutic interventions. In this chapter, we have explored some of the quantitative designs that can be used to address specific questions and the steps involved in undertaking quantitative research. Data collection for quantitative studies can be carried out in many ways, but the data must be quantifiable for analysis. Data analysis can be descriptive or inferential. The validity of study findings—that is, the degree to which they are free from bias—is an important concept in quantitative research.

Chapter review questions

- What is meant by quantitative research?
- What are some of the common quantitative designs used in nursing and midwifery research? How do they differ?
- What types of data do quantitative researchers collect?
- What are the main processes for quantitative data analysis?
- How are validity and reliability achieved in quantitative research?

Questions for discussion

- What are some possible applications for quantitative research in nursing and midwifery practice?
- How can nurses and midwives contribute to quantitative research knowledge and use?
- What are some of the challenges that might be faced in undertaking quantitative research?
- What strategies could be used to promote quantitative research in nursing and midwifery practice?

Questions for personal reflection

- How could quantitative research be employed to improve nursing or midwifery care?
- What have you learnt about quantitative research while working through this chapter?

Useful web resources

Catalogue of Bias, Centre for Evidence-based Medicine <https://catalogofbias.org/>.
Enhancing the Quality and Transparency of Health Research Network <www.equator-network.org>.

References and further reading

Beyea, S.C. & Slattery, M.J., 2013, 'Historical perspectives on evidence-based nursing', *Nursing Science Quarterly*, vol. 26, no. 2, pp. 152–155.

Capili, B., 2021a, 'Cross-sectional studies', *AJN, American Journal of Nursing*, vol. 121, no. 10, pp. 59–62.

Capili, B., 2021b, 'Selection and Implementation of outcome measurements', *AJN, American Journal of Nursing*, vol. 121, no. 8, pp. 63–67.

Curtis, A.C. & Keeler, C., 2021a, 'Measurement in nursing research', *AJN, American Journal of Nursing*, vol. 121, no. 6, pp. 56–60.

Curtis, A.C. & Keeler, C., 2021b, 'Sampling design in nursing research', *AJN, American Journal of Nursing*, vol. 121, no. 3, pp. 53–57.

Ekman, N., Taft, C., Moons, P., Makitalo, A., Bostrom, E. & Fors, A., 2020, 'A state-of-the-art review of direct observation tools for assessing competency in person-centred care', *International Journal of Nursing Studies*, vol. 109, p. 103634.

Field, A., 2017, *Discovering Statistics Using IBM SPSS Statistics*, 5th edn, London: Sage.

Hemming, K., Eldridge, S., Forbes, G., Weijer, C. & Taljaard, M., 2017, 'How to design efficient cluster randomised trials', *BMJ*, vol. 358, p. j3064. doi: 10.1136/bmj.j3064.

Hemming, K. & Taljaard, M., 2020, 'Reflection on modern methods: when is a stepped-wedge cluster randomized trial a good study design choice?', *International Journal of Epidemiology*, vol. 49, no. 3, pp. 1043–1052. doi: 10.1093/ije/dyaa077.

Hooper, R. & Eldridge, S.M., 2021, 'Cutting edge or blunt instrument: how to decide if a stepped wedge design is right for you', *BMJ Quality & Safety*, vol. 30, pp. 245–250.

Keeler, C. & Curtis, A.C., 2022, 'Case-control studies', *AJN, American Journal of Nursing*, vol. 122, no. 2, pp. 51–56.

Keeler, C. & Curtis, A.C., 2023, 'Introduction to statistical hypothesis testing in nursing research', *AJN, American Journal of Nursing*, vol. 123, no. 7, pp. 53–55.

Kuipers, Y.F., van Beeck, E., van den Berg, L. & Dijkhuizen, M., 2021, 'The comparison of the interpersonal action component of woman-centred care reported by healthy pregnant women in different sized practices in the Netherlands: A cross-sectional study', *Women & Birth: Journal of the Australian College of Midwives*, vol. 34, no. 4, pp. e376–e383.

Ruel, E., 2019, *100 Questions (and Answers) about Survey Research*, Thousand Oaks, CA: Sage.

Pallant, J., 2020, *SPSS Survival Manual: A Step by Step Guide to Data Analysis Using IBM SPSS*, 7th edn, London: Routledge.

Toivonen, M., Lehtonen, L., Ahlqvist-Bjorkroth, S. & Axelin, A., 2023, 'Effects of the close collaboration with parents intervention on the quality of family-centered care in NICUs', *Advances in Neonatal Care*, vol. 23, no. 3, pp. 281–289.

5 Understanding qualitative research approaches

Learning objectives

After working through this chapter, you should be able to:

- Define the term qualitative research
- Describe the benefits of qualitative research for nursing or midwifery practice
- Outline basic approaches to and differences between common qualitative research methodologies
- Outline the two main ways by which qualitative data analysis is performed
- Discuss strategies for ensuring quality and rigour in qualitative research

Key terms and concepts

Action research, audit trail, case study, confirmability, content analysis, credibility, data saturation, descriptive, discourse analysis, ethnography, fittingness, grounded theory, immersion, inductive, interpretive, methodology, paradigm, participatory research, phenomenology, qualitative, realities, thematic analysis, transferability, triangulation.

Case study overview

Jill is the unit manager for a busy medical-surgical unit. The ward has a strong philosophy around delivering person-centred care. However, lately, Jill has observed that nurses in the ward appear to be providing care that is not necessarily person-centred, and she is wondering whether this is related to their understanding of the philosophy and what it means. She wants to understand how the nurses perceive their implementation of person-centred care into their everyday work and whether there are other factors impacting on their abilities to deliver person-centred care. She decides that this kind of study requires a qualitative approach.

Chapter introduction

In the previous chapter, we explored quantitative methods for generating new knowledge and understandings. With quantitative approaches, the emphasis is on use of measurements and numbers. However, there are other types of data that are equally important for informing practice—that is, qualitative types. Qualitative research entails seeking understandings of human experiences and situations, primarily through using words and

DOI: 10.4324/9781003414476-7

text. This chapter focuses on qualitative research and how it applies to nursing and mid-wifery. One of the challenges in qualitative research is that there are many approaches and positions taken by researchers. While the chapter does not seek to offer insights into all of these, it aims to present an overview of the nature of qualitative research generally, with exploration of a few of the most commonly used approaches.

What is qualitative research?

Qualitative research is popular in nursing and midwifery as it involves close interaction with the people being studied, reflecting the levels of communication and personal interaction involved in professional nursing and midwifery work. It seeks to understand varied human realities and contexts. Qualitative research allows for rich understandings and can lead to development of theories that explain certain situations. Hence, it is well suited to nursing and midwifery practice, as they are both very interactive professions. It can also be useful when little is known about a particular topic and the researcher seeks to understand it better. Sometimes, qualitative research is used in mixed methods research to gain an understanding of a topic for which a quantitative survey can be subsequently developed. Alternatively, qualitative research may be used after a quantitative study to more fully understand the nature of a topic that cannot be explored in depth in a survey.

Differences between qualitative and quantitative research

As described in the previous chapter, quantitative research involves measuring and analysing relationships between variables—for example, through frequencies and other statistical analyses. Largely, quantitative research answers What? and How much? questions. On the other hand, qualitative research seeks understandings of processes and situations. It looks at how processes work and how individuals experience them.

The language of qualitative research is different from that of quantitative research and at times can seem overwhelming for a new reader. First, the person is seen as central to the whole process of qualitative research. Therefore, while people may be referred to as a group of *subjects* in quantitative research, in qualitative studies people who participate are known as *participants*. Second, there are multiple viewpoints, or **paradigms**, from which qualitative research is approached. **Interpretive research** attempts to interpret the experiences of people, while **participatory research** aims to work with participants to make change—participation is active—therefore, the relationship between the researcher and participants can differ.

While quantitative research believes there is one answer, or truth, qualitative research reflects the individual nature of human existence and explores social constructions. It believes that there are many ways to view the world and that each person's own truth is relevant and legitimate. Hence, qualitative research assumes multiple ways of seeing something. Consider, for example, patients' experiences of being in hospital: no two patients have completely the same experience, but each experience is real and relevant to the individual patient.

Given the different natures of qualitative research approaches, the data used are also different. Quantitative research is dependent on numbers and mathematical calculations. On the other hand, qualitative research collects mainly words or text. However, it may also draw on other types of data such as pictures and photographs.

Common qualitative approaches

There are many ways to go about doing qualitative research. The approach chosen is dependent on the research aim and question to be answered and upon the philosophical perspectives of the researcher. Our goal here is not to conduct an exhaustive discussion of each type but to have you appreciate that there are different approaches to conducting qualitative research. This will assist you as you read qualitative studies and try to make sense of them. There are many more qualitative approaches in nursing and midwifery than are covered in this chapter, but commonly used approaches include those discussed below.

Phenomenology

In phenomenology, the research is focused on understanding the meanings in the lived experiences of people in certain situations, or phenomena. This draws in the similarities and differences in people's experiences across similar situations. The researcher may *bracket*, or put aside, their own preconceived ideas on a situation. A range of specific approaches has evolved as phenomenology itself has evolved. In this chapter's case study, Jill may choose to use phenomenology to explore the experiences of staff in delivering patient-centred care. Even though she thinks she might know what the issues impacting on this are, she needs to put her own ideas aside and focus on those of her participants. Jill should not let her own preconceived ideas influence the analysis and interpretations of her findings.

Qualitative descriptive research

Sometimes, a researcher may choose to perform qualitative research without a strong philosophical underpinning so will carry out a descriptive qualitative study. This is similar to phenomenology in the way that the researcher seeks to provide a rich description of the topic or issue under study, but the researcher is less concerned with their own role in the study or in the underlying philosophical position. However, the researcher still needs to collect sufficient data to be able to draw sound conclusions. Qualitative description is often used in nursing and midwifery to explore clinical issues or give voice to patients or health professionals (Doyle et al., 2020). In our case study, if Jill were to employ a descriptive qualitative research approach to understanding the factors impacting on patient-centred care, she might choose to interview a number of staff members and analyse the interviews without a particularly focused approach.

Grounded theory

This approach explores social processes and how they work, by examining interactions between people. This allows a theory or model to be constructed that shows how processes operate and that is generated from, and grounded in, the data collected. Within grounded theory, there is a range of specific approaches that have evolved as grounded theory itself has evolved (Birks et al., 2019). In our case study, if Jill were to take a grounded theory approach, it would look different to that of other qualitative approaches. Jill would be focusing more on *how* staff actually went about providing patient-centred care in the ward, rather than just describing what happens or their personal experiences.

Research Tip 5.1   Common qualitative approaches used in nursing and midwifery

Action research	Works with individuals or groups to make, implement and evaluate changes (see Chapter 8)
Case study	Examines the complexities of unique stories to explore a particular phenomenon
Discourse analysis	Examines social and political factors that shape the development of certain practices or circumstances
Ethnography	Examines cultural patterns existing in a particular group
Ethnomethodology	Examines the ways in which people feel, understand and explain their world
Grounded theory	Examines social processes and how they work in certain situations
Historical research	Examines the historical development of a particular concept or situation
Narrative research	Explores the experiences of people through the stories they tell
Phenomenology	Examines the lived experiences of individuals in certain situations

Activity 5.1   Exploring a qualitative research approach

1 Choose one qualitative research approach and do some reading about its origins and evolution.
2 Search for one or two research studies that have used that methodology.
3 Summarise the key aspects of the methodology.

Questions for consideration

• How have the researchers in your chosen studies used the methodology?
• Can you think of a study where you could use that particular methodology?

Steps in undertaking a qualitative research study

Qualitative research studies follow similar steps to quantitative studies—that is, identifying a problem or issue, conducting an initial literature review, developing a research question, identifying the population under study, considering the ethical aspects in conducting the study, collecting data, analysing data and then reporting the findings. However, there are some differences in how the research question is framed, the actual ethical considerations and how the data are collected, analysed and reported. (Ethical considerations are covered in more detail in Chapter 7.)

Developing a qualitative research question

Unlike quantitative research, which seeks to quantify or connect cause and effect, qualitative research seeks to understand a particular topic or issue in more depth. Developing a qualitative research question requires great consideration to ensure that it will actually answer the identified problem or issue. A sound research question is clear, specific and able to be researched. Unlike quantitative research questions, qualitative research questions are open ended in nature. The aim is to not limit what might be found and to yield large amounts of textual or observational data. Closed-ended questions do not facilitate the acquisition of such data.

In our case study, Jill wants to understand what staff understand by the concept of person-centred care and what impacts on their ability to deliver such care. Appropriately descriptive qualitative questions might include the following:

- What are nurses' understandings of person-centred care?
- What factors impact on nurses' abilities to deliver person-centred care, and in what ways?
- How do nurses perceive their delivery of person-centred care in the ward?

If Jill wants to use a particular qualitative approach, she may use slightly more refined questions:

- For a **phenomenological** study, she might ask: What are the nurses' lived experiences of delivering person-centred care in the ward?
- If it was a **grounded theory** study, she might ask: How do nurses deliver person-centred care in the ward?
- If she chose a **discourse analysis,** the question might be: What shapes the way in which nurses deliver patient-centred care in the ward?

It is important for the question to align with the type of qualitative approach used. The goal is to keep the question broad, in order to access the types of data required. Activity 5.2 provides an opportunity to develop research questions aligned to a specific approach.

Collecting qualitative data

There are many approaches to collecting qualitative data, including interviews, observations of people in their natural environments, written text sources such as newspapers, documents and records, photographs and other pictures and social media posts. For example, a phenomenological researcher wanting to understand the patient experience of living with chronic back pain might choose to do one-on-one interviews with patients to record their individual experiences. The grounded theory researcher might choose to

---

Activity 5.2   Exploring person-centred care qualitatively

Imagine you want to explore nursing students' experiences of delivering person-centred care in their clinical placements. Write a short, clear research question that could be asked for each of the following research approaches:

- Descriptive qualitative
- Phenomenology
- Grounded theory

explore the processes by which the person copes with their chronic pain, and then develop a model by which patients live with such conditions, so might use a combination of interviews and observations of people in their homes. Common data collection methods in qualitative research include the following:

- **Interviews** Most often, interviews are performed one to one, that is, between the researcher and the person being researched. The researcher may use very structured or semi-structured interview questions, depending on the underlying research approach being taken. Interviews are usually audio-recorded, transcribed verbatim (word for word) and then analysed.
- **Focus groups** These are a type of interview conducted with a group of people at the same time. They give participants the opportunity to explore collective experiences through sharing and building on ideas. Focus groups normally contain from two to ten participants. Like individual interviews, they are usually audio-recorded and transcribed later for analysis. However, there may also be an observer in the room taking field notes—for example, about the interaction of participants.
- **Participant observation** This involves observing participants in the research setting; the researcher usually takes field notes recording their observations for later analysis.
- **Photovoice** This is a newer, but increasingly popular, qualitative research approach, particularly in participatory research, such as action research. It employs the use of photographs to present viewpoints from participants' unique worlds.
- **Surveys** Qualitative survey responses commonly seek open-ended responses rather than closed-ended responses that can be analysed using statistics.

In our case study, it is evident that Jill has a number of options for collecting the data needed to answer her research question. She could do individual interviews, run focus groups with staff, observe staff in their practice or ask them to document their ideas about patient-centred care delivery. Therefore, Jill will need to be clear about her research approach and how best to answer her research question. What would you suggest?

Sourcing research participants and collecting data

Unlike quantitative research, qualitative studies use small samples. Participants for these studies are usually chosen through convenience or **purposive sampling**. The qualitative researcher does not seek to generalise their findings to other populations, and they look for people who can provide the specific information that will help them answer their research question and understand the phenomenon they are studying.

Research Tip 5.2   Potential data sources for qualitative research

Audio	Interviews, focus groups, podcasts
Electronic	Internet, social media posts
Visual	Pictures, video footage, photographs, observation
Written	Newspapers, magazines, reports, documents, diaries, letters

---

Activity 5.3   Planning qualitative research

Choose one of the research questions you designed in Activity 5.2.

Questions for consideration
- How might you source the data needed to answer the question?
- Who might your participants be?
- What might be the best method or methods to access the data?

In seeking out suitable participants, qualitative researchers often use an approach known as **snowball sampling**. This involves using recommendations for suitable participants from people already participating in the research: the sampling rolls on like a snowball.

Theoretical sampling is a technique used in grounded theory approaches. The process of sampling continues until the theory being generated is completed. This approach is used to decide where, when and how to collect the next tranche of data (Birks et al., 2019).

Qualitative research does not have tight sample-size boundaries such as those associated with quantitative methods. At the point of **data saturation**—when the researcher is not obtaining any new data or new insights into the phenomenon being studied—they need to make the decision to stop collecting data. Recently, the concept of **information power** has emerged as an alternative to data saturation. This concept considers the study aim, sample specificity, use of established theory, quality of dialogue and the strategy used for analysis to determine if a qualitative study sample is sufficient for drawing sound conclusions (Malterud et al., 2016). These are particularly important concepts, as failure to achieve data saturation or information power may negatively impact on the overall conclusions drawn and strength of the study findings. Hence, in evaluating qualitative research, it is important to determine if data saturation or information power have been achieved.

Returning to our chapter case study, let's consider how Jill decides to proceed with her qualitative research. Following a great deal of consideration, Jill decides to undertake a descriptive qualitative study to really understand the staff perceptions and understandings of person-centred care. Her research aim is to examine their understandings of person-centred care. In line with that, she develops her research question: *What are nurses' understandings of person-centred care?* Jill then decides that the most appropriate data collection method is semi-structured interview. Her **interview schedule** contains two key guiding questions but allows sufficient space for discussion to proceed in other directions. The key questions are:

- What do you understand by the term *person-centred care*?
- How do you perceive that person-centred care is provided in your clinical setting?

Jill opts to employ purposive sampling, as she plans to target a specific group of participants—that is, the staff working on the ward. She realises that there may not be enough participants on her ward to enable her to achieve data saturation so considers employing snowball sampling, with her initial participants recommending other potential participants.

Activity 5.4   Collecting qualitative data

Choose one of the research questions you designed in Activity 5.2.

Questions for consideration
- Where would you find the right participants to provide data for the research?
- What sampling processes would you employ?
- Where would be the best place to collect the data?
- When would you stop the data collection process?

Managing and analysing qualitative data

When and how the process of data analysis begins depends on the research approach adopted. For example, in some approaches, all the data are collected before analysis begins. In others, such as grounded theory research, analysis occurs throughout the data collection, as data are constantly compared in order to build a theory.

Qualitative research can generate immense amounts of data, which the researcher needs to manage. Initially, the researcher needs to *immerse* themselves into the data to become familiar with their contents and meaning. **Data immersion** may require several readings of transcripts and multiple listenings to recordings. It is imperative that the researcher ensure the participants' intended meanings are not lost.

There are many ways to approach the analysis of qualitative data. Most of these involve **coding** and then categorising data, which require a significant investment of time to do accurately. Coding involves working through each line or paragraph, depending on the overall approach, for data that address the research question. These segments of data are then marked, or coded. In the next step, codes are arranged into groups of similar meanings, where they can be further grouped into broad categories, which may have associated subcategories.

In some research approaches, there are specific processes for coding data. For example, in grounded theory there are different levels of coding: initial coding with early data collected; intermediate coding, known as *selective, axial* or *focused coding*, where categories and theory are emerging and advanced coding, where there is finalising of the theory (Mills et al., 2014).

The two main approaches to data analysis reported in the nursing and midwifery research literature are *thematic analysis* and *content analysis*. Often, they are incorrectly interchanged, but they are different.

Thematic analysis

Thematic analysis involves taking an **inductive approach** to find meanings from data. There are many described approaches to undertaking thematic analysis. One common approach is described by Braun and Clarke (2006, p. 87) in a six-step process:

1 The researcher first familiarises themself with the data.
2 Next, initial codes are generated.

3 From the initial codes, the researcher searches to find patterns of similar ideas—that is, **themes**.
4 From this, the themes emerging from the dataset are reviewed and refined.
5 Next, each of the themes is defined and given a title or name.
6 Finally, the themes are reported.

Content analysis

There are various understandings as to what constitutes content analysis. It is considered more deductive in nature than thematic analysis, seeking to draw descriptive conclusions from the data, rather than broad understandings (Crowe et al., 2015). Content analysis is often suited to smaller qualitative datasets, such as those obtained through open-ended survey questions where there is insufficient data to create themes through thematic analysis.

In some approaches to content analysis, qualitative data may be quantified. Polgar and Thomas (2019) describe such an approach whereby the meaningful pieces of text, particularly words or key terms, are counted and described in number format. They suggest that statistical analysis can then be applied to the data and hypotheses tested.

The researcher needs to determine whether they are going to approach data analysis manually, by labelling or highlighting text, or using computer-assisted qualitative data analysis, or CAQDAS. There are many software programs available to assist researchers, such as NVivo and ATLAS.ti. While still requiring the researcher to code data segments, these programs facilitate searching and grouping of data into patterns or categories.

In our case study, Jill undertakes ten semi-structured interviews. Each is audio-recorded and lasts between 48 and 56 minutes. She chooses to transcribe them herself, as she does not have the funding to send them to a professional transcriber. In total, she ends up with 300 pages of double-spaced text. In line with her theoretical approach, Jill chooses to use thematic analysis and finds two key themes emerging. Under each theme, there emerge sub-themes, as follows:

> Theme 1: The nature of person-centred care in the ward
>   Sub-theme: How person-centred care is being delivered
>   Sub-theme: Factors impacting on person-centred care delivery
>   Theme 2: Staff readiness for person-centred care
>   Sub-theme: Understandings of person-centred care and providing such care
>   Sub-theme: Educational preparation of staff
>   Sub-theme: Attitudes surrounding person-centred care

Research Example 5.1   Using qualitative descriptive research to study woman-centred midwifery care during the COVID-19 pandemic

Woman-centred care is a fundamental underpinning to midwifery practice. Stulz et al. (2022) undertook a qualitative study with 26 Australian midwives to explore how the pandemic impacted on their delivery of woman-centred care and what had been learned during this time. The researchers conducted in-depth interviews via telephone or online platforms and interviews lasted between 20 and 70 minutes in duration. Thematic analysis was used from which two overarching themes, *COVID-19 causing chaos* and *Keeping the woman at the centre of care*, emerged. The first them included three sub-themes: *quickly evolving situation, challenges to provide care* and *affecting women and families*. The second theme comprised three sub-themes: *trying to keep it normal, bending the rules and pushing the boundaries, and quality time for the woman, baby, and family unit.* The researchers concluded that during the pandemic midwives worked to ensure woman-centred care continued and enabling quality midwifery care was delivered.

Stulz, V.M., Bradfield, Z., Cummins, A., Catling, C., Sweet, L., McInnes, R., McLaughlin, K., Taylor, J., Hartz, D. & Sheehan, A., 2022, 'Midwives providing woman-centred care during the COVID-19 pandemic in Australia: A national qualitative study', *Women and Birth*, vol. 35, pp. 475–483.

Questions for consideration

- Why was qualitative description an appropriate research approach for this study?
- What do the findings tell about midwives' experiences?
- How might the findings be used in midwifery practice?

Research Example 5.2   Using a qualitative descriptive approach to study person-centred care

Person-centred care is important for ensuring continuity of effective health care. A study by Kim and Kim (2023) used a qualitative descriptive approach to describe nursing students' experiences of barriers to the implementation of person-centred care in clinical settings in South Korea. To explore this issue, the researchers conducted semi-structured individual interviews with 17 nursing students. Their interview schedule comprised seven key questions. Interviews lasted between 14 and 36 minutes. Data were analysed using inductive content analysis using ATLAS.ti 8.2. From the analysis, five categories emerged that described their experiences: *busyness* relating to workforce shortages and excessive workloads, *educational challenges* due to lack of education around person-centred care, *lack of awareness* of person-centred care by nurses and patients, *lack of relationship building* with patients and *lack of policy approaches* within institutions to guide the delivery of person-centred care.

Kim, S. & Kim, M., 2023, 'Nursing students' experiences and perceptions of barriers to the implementation of person-centred care in clinical settings: A qualitative study', Nursing Open, vol. 10, pp. 1889–1899.

Questions for consideration

- Why was a descriptive qualitative research approach appropriate for this study?
- What do the findings tell about delivery of person-centred care in practice?
- How might the findings be applied to nursing practice?

Ensuring quality of qualitative research

Qualitative research has been criticised as not being rigorous in its approaches. While that may be true of some qualitative research, there are, as with quantitative research, methods that researchers should employ to enhance the accuracy of the conclusions they draw. Key concepts include: *data saturation, credibility, fittingness (transferability), dependability, triangulation* and *confirmability*. In addition to these concepts, it is vital that qualitative researchers ensure that their research approach and design are consistent with their overarching philosophical approach. This means that their research question, sampling, data collection methods, data analysis and reporting should all be in line with the chosen approach.

Credibility

Credibility is achieved when the interpretations and conclusions drawn by the researcher are truly reflective of the views and details presented by the participants. **Member checking** is one way in which credibility can be assessed: Using this, the researcher returns to participants to check that the interpretations represent their experiences accurately. This process can be undertaken verbally or by providing a written summary to participants (Candela, 2019).

Fittingness

Fittingness, also known as **transferability,** is the degree to which research findings can be transferred and have similar meanings, to other, similar populations. The researcher cannot measure this; rather, only users of the research can do so (Lincoln & Guba, 1985). In reporting on fittingness, researchers generally recognise that their findings are not generalisable but may have meaning or resonance with others in similar situations.

Dependability

Dependability is the consistency of findings in other, similar conditions. **Triangulation** is one way to promote research dependability, through the use of multiple methods or data sources that the researcher can verify and from which they can draw accurate conclusions. Moon (2019) identifies four types of triangulation that may be used to ensure the dependability of qualitative research:

1 **Method triangulation** A combination of data collection methods is used (such as interviews, observations, field notes and journaling) within one study.
2 **Investigator triangulation** More than one researcher undertakes the interpretation of data and drawing of conclusions.
3 **Theory triangulation** More than one theory is employed in analysing and interpreting data, assisting with supporting the conclusions drawn.
4 **Data source triangulation** Data are drawn from a range of sources (such as different types of participants) to ensure that multiple perspectives are captured.

Previously in this chapter, we discussed the concept of data saturation—that is considered the point at which no new data are emerging. Ensuring sufficient participation is particularly important for ensuring that data are complete and that key aspects of a phenomenon have not been left out of the final interpretations.

Confirmability

Confirmability refers to the degree to which the findings represent the participants' responses and viewpoints. In order to achieve confirmability, reporting of findings should use rich verbatim text quotes from participants that reinforce conclusions drawn (Stenfors et al., 2020). Documentation of the research process is also an important consideration with regard to confirmability. Throughout the research process, researchers should maintain an audit trail, documenting the steps taken and decisions made, that could be followed by another researcher (Johnson et al., 2020).

Reporting findings

While there is no specific approach to reporting qualitative findings, it is important to consider who the intended audience is and to write with them in mind, and to ensure the theoretical framework is in line with the employed methodology throughout. There are numerous elements that need to be included in the research report:

- **Background** Introduction to the study and what was already known about the topic.
- **Paradigm and theoretical framework** The philosophy underpinning the study.
- **Research problem, research aim and research question** The problem that the research is exploring, what the research aims to do, and the question guiding the study.
- **Method** Details of the method chosen—for example, if interviews were employed, the interview schedule, the number conducted, their setting and duration, how they were recorded and transcribed; if observations were employed, where they were conducted, the number conducted and the types of data collected.
- **Participants** Details about participants and how they were recruited into the study.
- **Ethical considerations** Steps taken to manage potential ethical issues, and details of approval by Human Research Ethics Committee.
- **Data analysis** Outline of selected approach and step-by-step description of how analysis was performed.
- **Trustworthiness and rigour** Details of processes by which these were managed in regard to findings, with reference to credibility, transferability, dependability, confirmability and data saturation.
- **Findings** Presented as themes or categories, which may also contain sub-themes or subcategories; all conclusions evidenced through inclusion of appropriate participant quotations that clearly support each claim made; reflect views from a range of participants.

Chapter summary

Qualitative research is commonly performed in nursing and midwifery. It reflects the nature of human experience with which nurses and midwives continually engage and has many differences to quantitative approaches. There are various ways to do qualitative research, depending on the research aim and question. In this chapter, we have explored common qualitative approaches used in nursing and midwifery research, though many others can be utilised. Varied types of data can be used in qualitative research and can be analysed using methods such as thematic and content analysis, while rigour and trustworthiness can be achieved through a range of strategies.

Activity 5.5   Analysing a qualitative research report

1 Search for a qualitative research paper on a topic that is of interest to you.
2 Carefully review the methods section. Note the strategies used by the researcher to ensure the quality of their findings.
3 Examine the way in which the research is reported through the paper.

Questions for consideration

• Were the quality-control strategies sufficiently rigorous?
• Were there other strategies that could have been employed to enhance their rigour?
• Does the paper clearly describe the necessary details of the research?
• Are there any research components missing from the paper?
• What are the strengths of the report?

Chapter review questions

• What is meant by qualitative research?
• What are some of the common qualitative approaches used in nursing and midwifery research? How do they differ?
• What types of data do qualitative researchers collect?
• What are the main processes for qualitative data analysis?
• How is rigour achieved in qualitative research?

Questions for discussion

• What are some possible applications for qualitative research to nursing and/or midwifery practice?
• How can nurses and midwives contribute to qualitative research knowledge and use?
• What are some of the challenges that might be faced in undertaking qualitative research?
• What strategies could be used to promote qualitative research in nursing and midwifery practice?

Questions for personal reflection

• How could qualitative research be employed to improve nursing or midwifery care?
• What have you learnt about qualitative research while working through this chapter?

Useful web resources

Association for Qualitative Research <https://www.aqr.org.uk/>.

References and further reading

Adamson, E., Pow, J., Houston, F. & Redpath, P., 2016, 'Exploring the experiences of patients attending day hospitals in the rural Scotland: Capturing the patient's voice', *Journal of Clinical Nursing*, vol. 26, pp. 3044–3055.

Atchan, M., Davis, D. & Foureur, M., 2016, 'A methodological review of qualitative case study methodology in midwifery research', *Journal of Advanced Nursing*, vol. 72, no. 10, pp. 2259–2271.

Beardsmore, E. & McSherry, R., 2017, 'Healthcare workers' perceptions of organisation culture and the impact on the delivery of compassionate quality care', *Journal of Research in Nursing*, vol. 22, no. 1–2, pp. 42–56.

Birks, M., Hoare, K. & Mills, J., 2019. 'Grounded theory: The FAQs', *International Journal of Qualitative Methods*, vol. 18, pp. 1–7. doi: 10.1177/160940691982535.

Braun, V. & Clarke, V., 2006, 'Using thematic analysis in psychology', *Qualitative Research in Psychology*, vol. 3, no. 2, pp. 77–101.

Candela, A.G., 2019, 'Exploring the function of member checking', *The Qualitative Report*, vol. 24, no. 3, pp. 619–628.

Charmaz, K. & Thornberg, R., 2021, 'The pursuit of quality in grounded theory', *Qualitative Research in Psychology*, vol. 18, no. 3, pp. 305–327.

Coyne, E., Grafton, E. & Reid, A., 2016, 'Strategies to successfully recruit and engage clinical nurses as participants in qualitative clinical research', *Contemporary Nurse*, vol. 52, no. 6, pp. 669–676.

Crowe, M., Inder, M., & Porter, R., 2015, 'Conducting qualitative research in mental health: Thematic and content analysis', *Australian & New Zealand Journal of Psychiatry*, vol. 49, no. 7, pp. 616–623.

Cypress, B., 2022, 'Qualitative research methods: A phenomenological focus', *Dimensions of Critical Care Nursing*, vol. 37, no. 6, pp. 302–309.

Denzin, N.K., 1978, *The Research Act: A Theoretical Introduction to Sociological Methods*, 2nd edn, New York: McGraw-Hill.

Doyle, L., McCabe, C., Keogh, B., Brady, A. & McCann, M., 2020, 'An overview of the qualitative descriptive design within nursing research', *Journal of Research in Nursing*, vol. 25, no. 5, pp. 443–455.

Florczak, K.L., 2017, 'Adding to the truth of the matter: The case for qualitative research', *Nursing Science Quarterly*, vol. 30, no. 4, pp. 296–299.

Houghton, C., Casey, D. & Smyth, S., 2017, 'Selection, collection and analysis as sources of evidence in case study research', *Nurse Researcher*, vol. 24, no. 4, pp. 36–41.

Johnson, J.L., Adkins, D. & Chauvin, S., 2020, 'Qualitative research in pharmacy education: A review of the quality indicators of rigor in qualitative research', *American Journal of Pharmaceutical Education*, vol. 84, no. 1, article 7120.

Kim, S. & Kim, M., 2023, 'Nursing students' experiences and perceptions of barriers to the implementation of person-centred care in clinical settings: A qualitative study', *Nursing Open*, vol. 10, pp. 1889–1899.

Liebenberg, L., 2018, 'Thinking critically about photovoice: Achieving empowerment and social change', *International Journal of Qualitative Methods*, vol. 17, no. 1. doi: 10.1177/1609406918757631.

Lincoln, Y.S. & Guba, E., 1985, *Naturalistic Inquiry*, Beverly Hills, CA: Sage.

Malterud, K., Siersma, V.D. & Guassora, A.D. 2016, 'Sample size in qualitative interview studies: Guided by information power', *Qualitative Health Research*, vol. 26, no. 13, pp. 1753–1760.

Mayan, M.J., 2023, *Essentials of Qualitative Inquiry*, 2nd edn, New York: Routledge.

Mills, J., Birks, M. & Hoare, K., 2014, 'Grounded theory', in J. Mills & M. Birks (eds), *Qualitative Methodology: A Practical Guide*, London: Sage, pp. 107–121.

Moon, M.D., 2019, 'Triangulation: A method to increase validity, reliability, and legitimation in clinical research', *Journal of Emergency Nursing*, vol. 45, no. 1, pp. 103–105.

Polgar, S. & Thomas, S., 2019, *Introduction to Research in the Health Sciences*, 7th edn, Edinburgh: Churchill Livingstone Elsevier.

Ryan, G.S., 2017, 'An introduction to the origins, history and principles of ethnography', *Nurse Researcher*, vol. 24, no. 4, pp. 15–21.

Stenfors, T., Kajamaa, A. & Bennett, D., 2020, 'How to … assess the quality of qualitative research', *The Clinical Teacher*, vol. 17, pp. 596–599.

Streubert, H.J. & Carpenter, D.R., 2011, *Qualitative Research in Nursing: Advancing the Humanistic Imperative*, Philadelphia, PA: Wolters Kluwer.

Stulz, V.M., Bradfield, Z., Cummins, A., Catling, C., Sweet, L., McInnes, R., McLaughlin, K., Taylor, J., Hartz, D. & Sheehan, A., 2022, 'Midwives providing woman-centred care during the COVID-19 pandemic in Australia: A national qualitative study', *Women and Birth*, vol. 35, pp. 475–483.

Turner, C. & Astin, F., 2021, 'Grounded theory: What makes a grounded theory study?', *European Journal of Cardiovascular Nursing*, vol. 20, pp. 285–289.

Wolf, A., 2017, 'What qualitative research can do for you: Deriving solutions and interventions from qualitative findings', *Journal of Emergency Nursing*, vol. 43, no. 5, pp. 484–485.

Section 3

How Do I Critically Evaluate Research Studies?

Critique involves a detailed process of evaluation of research. It is paramount for nurses and midwives to ensure that the best possible evidence is being used in practice. The implementation of substandard or poorly designed research outcomes could lead to poor and inappropriate care delivery and have detrimental outcomes for those being cared for. This section centres on how to approach critical research reviews.

Chapter 6 focuses on the steps involved in making judgements about the quality of published research. It begins by looking at how to approach critiquing an individual research report. The second part of the chapter presents two increasingly popular types of critical literature reviews—namely, the scoping review and the systematic review, which involve analysing a group of research studies on a topic.

Chapter 7 focuses on ethical considerations in human research. Understanding these is crucial to being able to fully critique practical aspects of research approaches. It involves how ethical principles apply to research, as well as the roles of Human Research Ethics Committees and researchers with regard to the ethical conduct of research.

DOI: 10.4324/9781003414476-8

6   Critiquing research

DOI: 10.4324/9781003414476-9

Learning objectives

After working through this chapter, you should be able to:

- Discuss what is meant by *critique* of a research study
- Outline the steps involved in undertaking a critique of research
- Discuss ways in which author and journal quality can be evaluated
- Discuss the roles of systematic and scoping reviews in research critique
- Explain the differences between systematic and scoping reviews

Key terms and concepts

Critique, H-index, impact factor, journal quality, predatory journals, quartile ranking, research quality, scoping review, systematic review.

Case study overview

Alice is a clinical nurse specialist who is interested in the effectiveness of vital signs monitoring in her ward. She suspects that nurses on the ward are missing key changes in patients' conditions. Knowing that subtle changes can indicate early deterioration in a patient's status, she is concerned that early changes in vital signs are not being detected and deterioration is only being identified when it is well established.

Chapter introduction

Over the past decade, the volume of available research to inform nursing and midwifery practice has exploded and continues to grow every day. This makes it difficult to keep up-to-date with evidence to support best clinical practice. Unfortunately, the quality of the available research can vary significantly, so the ability to critique it becomes very important. In this chapter, we will work through the process of critiquing research studies. In the second half of the chapter, we will explore some structured review approaches to critiquing bodies of research that are becoming popular in nursing and midwifery—namely, the systematic review and scoping review—as means of managing the large body of research that exists in any one topic area.

Critiquing and evaluating research quality

The ability to **critique** research is important for students at both undergraduate and postgraduate levels. Qualified nurses and midwives also need this ability, as they may be invited to provide peer-reviewed critique of research submitted for consideration for publication in journals. Furthermore, healthcare professionals need to be able to effectively critique research studies to ensure that they are delivering best practice to the people they care for and that they are not implementing practice interventions based on poorly designed research. Many people incorrectly think of *critique* as criticising or finding faults in a work. While this may happen in the process, proper critique involves taking an objective view in assessing a research study to identify its strengths and weaknesses and how the findings apply to practice.

   Effective critique of research is appropriately complex. Regardless of whether you are reviewing papers for an assignment or a literature review, there are some key steps in critiquing and evaluating the quality of published research studies.

Title

The title should clearly indicate what the paper is about and should be short. Often, journals limit the number of words contained in titles, by requiring them to be no more than ten words long, for example. In many journals, the type of research study being reported on is also included in the title. Questions to ask of the title include:

* Does it indicate what the paper is about?
* Does it reflect the research undertaken?
* Is it clear and appropriately written?

Author

Details about the author (or authors) are essential considerations. It is important to assess whether the researcher (or researchers) is affiliated with a reputable institution, such as a hospital or university. In addition, where possible, it is good to explore whether they have a qualification in which they have learnt research skills, such as a masters by research or Doctor of Philosophy (PhD). One measure of a researcher's output is the **h-index**, which measures the number of citations received by a researcher, according to their most-cited articles. For example, a researcher who has been cited ten or more times in ten publications has an h-index of 10. The higher the h-index, the better. In nursing and midwifery, H-indexes are relatively low compared to other fields. McKenna et al. (2017) analysed the research publication performance of Australian nursing and midwifery professors and found the median h-index was 14 for professors and seven for associate professors. Questions to consider about the author include:

* Are they affiliated with a reputable institution?
* Do they have research qualifications?
* What is their h-index?

Journal

There is great diversity in the quality of journals themselves. Evaluating them is complex but important in assessing the overall quality of the research being published. It is likely that better journals publish better quality research papers. There are many bogus journals, known as **predatory journals**, which appear legitimate and reputable but are anything but. Often, these so-called journals do not have appropriate peer review (review by peers in the relevant field) processes in place for reviewing manuscripts and no editorial boards to monitor journal quality; they exist merely to make money out of inexperienced researchers. They often publish one or two volumes then disappear with the work of a researcher whose own long-term credibility is threatened by publishing with them (Darbyshire et al., 2017). Predatory publishers may publish work that credible journals would not and that may be based on flawed research processes. The ability to critique journal quality is, therefore, paramount to ensuring that only high-quality research is being implemented into clinical practice.

Journal quality can be assessed in a variety of ways. First, the journal should have a credible editor in charge. Therefore, it is worth finding out a bit about the editor, which can be done easily. They should be supported by an editorial board, associate editors or both. Second, the journal should have a sound, documented process for managing peer review of manuscripts. Oermann et al. (2020) suggest that promise of rapid review and publication should be a red flag for authors, as quality reviews take some time to complete. Third, the journal should be published by a credible organisation—usually a recognised publisher or a professional institution. Journals that are sound will be members of the Committee on Publication Ethics (or COPE) and in the case of nursing and midwifery should also be on the International Academy of Nursing Editors (or INANE) journal listing.

The best of the credible journals can be determined using additional strategies to rank them on a range of criteria; the two most commonly used are quartile ranking and impact factor. **Quartile ranking** orders all of the journals in a discipline according to quality criteria and then groups them into the top 25% (Q1), second 25% (Q2), third 25% (Q3) and bottom 25% (Q4). The best journals, therefore, are those in Q1, which constitutes the top 25% for that field. The SCImago Journal & Country Rank (or SJR) indicator takes this approach and is easily accessible. The **impact factor** measures the average citations of papers from a particular journal. For example, if a journal has an impact factor of 1.35, this indicates that on average each paper published in that journal is cited by other papers 1.35 times. The higher the impact factor, the higher the impact and quality of the journal. Again, in nursing and midwifery, impact factors are lower than in other disciplines. In 2022, nursing impact factors ranged from 8.1 (for the *International Journal of Nursing Studies*) to 0.1. It is important to note that not all credible journals have an impact factor, as it can take many years to qualify. Impact factor information can be sourced in various places, such as journal websites; at the International Scientific Institute's Journal Impact Factor List (see Research Tip 6.1); and through databases accessible through your library, such as Scopus and Web of Science. As will be clear now, evaluating the quality of a journal is complex but important in assessing the overall quality of the research being published. Questions to ask of a journal include:

- Is it a reputable journal?
- What types of papers does it publish?
- Does it have a recognised editor and editorial board?
- Is it published on listings of credible journals?
- What is its quartile ranking?
- What is its impact factor (if applicable)?

Research Tip 6.1 Places to check for journal credibility

- Databases like Scopus or Web of Science, which should be accessible through your institution's library
- Directory of Open Access Journals <https://doaj.org>
- International Academy of Nursing Editors' Directory of Nursing Journals <https://nursingeditors.com/journals-directory/>
- International Scientific Institute's Journal Impact Factor List <www.scijournal.org>
- SCImago Journal & Country Rank <www.scimagojr.com>

Abstract

The abstract is a short summary of the paper, around 100 to 300 words in length depending on the journal. From it, you should get a sense of the whole study. It should provide an overview of the background to the study; the aim or problem being researched; the research design, data collection and data analysis approaches; key findings and recommendations or implications for practice. Questions to ask of the abstract include:

- Does it provide an overview of how the whole study was conducted?
- Does it provide recommendations or implications for practice?

Introduction and background literature review

This section tells you a lot about the planning undertaken for the research and the current knowledge in the field being researched. It should be focused and demonstrate the deficits or gaps in existing research, justifying why the current study is needed. Questions to ask about the introduction and background literature review include:

- Do they demonstrate a sound understanding and overview of the topic and what is already known?
- Are all the key previous studies mentioned?
- Are the sources used original, that is, primary sources?
- Is information taken from other studies used out of its original context?
- Is there critical review of the literature?
- Does the review demonstrate a gap in existing knowledge?
- Is the problem clearly identified?

Methodology

The methodology presents the theoretical framework underpinning the research study. In qualitative studies, this may include an overview of a philosophical position, such as phenomenology or grounded theory. It presents the lens through which the study was conducted, such as how the data were collected and analysed. Questions to ask of the methodology include:

- Is the aim of the study clearly stated?
- Is the theoretical approach consistent with the study aim?
- For qualitative studies, is the underlying philosophical position described?

Study design

The study design should align directly with the chosen methodology and the research aim or question and the data collection methods should be described. The section should demonstrate how rigour was achieved in the research process. Research tools should be described in detail. How this is done depends largely on the type of study being reported. For example, if a questionnaire was used, it would be important to understand how it was developed and validated and, if it was a new tool, piloted. If qualitative interviews were used, the interview guide should be presented, listing the key interview questions and highlighting how the research aim or question was being addressed. In addition, the study participants should be described in detail including how they were selected for inclusion in the study, how they were recruited to the study and what their participation entailed. Questions to ask about the study design include:

- Is the research design consistent with the research aim?
- Is the design clearly explained and recognisable?
- Are participants well described?
- Who was included and who was excluded?
- How were participants sampled and recruited?
- Is the sample size sufficient to draw meaningful conclusions?
- Are the research instruments appropriate to answer the research question?
- Are these instruments valid and reliable?
- Was a pilot study conducted?

Ethical considerations

Ethical considerations with regard to research on humans are covered in detail in Chapter 7. Any research that involves humans must adhere to strict guidelines and processes to ensure that the rights and safety of the person are upheld throughout. All researchers engaging in research are expected to describe the steps taken to ensure that these are managed appropriately. Questions that need to be posed with regard to this aspect include:

- Are relevant ethical considerations, such as informed consent, confidentiality and data security, discussed?
- Were potential ethical issues appropriately managed?
- Is there a statement indicating that the study was approved by a Human Research Ethics Committee?

Data collection

Each of the data collection methods used in the study needs to be fully described. If using questionnaires, researchers need to describe how these were developed, how they were distributed and managed. If using interviews, the questions guiding the interviews should be presented. The time at which data were collected is also important; if data are old, findings may be irrelevant to current practice. Furthermore, the setting in which the data were collected may not be applicable to local practice settings, so implementation in other places may not be appropriate. Questions to ask about data collection include:

- When and where were the data collected?
- Were the data collection methods appropriate for the chosen methodology and research question?
- If appropriate, how were participants assigned to groups?
- Are the data collection methods justified by the authors?

Data analysis

In this section, the processes by which data were managed and analysed need to be fully explained. For statistical data, the tests conducted on them should be outlined, and these tests need to be clearly appropriate for types of data obtained. For qualitative data, how they were coded and grouped also requires clear description. Questions to ask about data analysis include:

- Are the processes by which the data were analysed fully explained?
- Were these processes appropriate for the chosen methodology and research design?
- For quantitative research, were the appropriate statistical tests performed? Were they accurate? Are they appropriately presented?
- For qualitative research, is the way in which data were managed well explained?
- Is the presentation of findings consistent with the chosen methodology?
- How were findings verified?

Interpretation of results

Interpretation of results is usually included in the discussion section of the research report. The findings of the study are positioned in the context of what is already known about the topic, showing how the new findings contribute to the existing body of knowledge. Issues arising or limitations in the study need to be fully and clearly described, and there should be recommendations for future research, practice or education. Questions to ask about the interpretation of results include:

- Did the study answer the research question or aim?
- Are the researcher's conclusions supported by the findings?
- Are the findings generalisable? If not, are they representative of the broader population?
- Has any potential bias been identified?
- Are the limitations of the study explained? Are they sufficient?
- Are implications and recommendations for practice or future research presented?
- What new questions have emerged?
- Is the new knowledge generated made explicit?

Conflicts of interest

Research should be free of any potential bias. It is important to examine whether there are potential areas where the researchers may have experienced conflicts of interest. Funding is one area where this may arise, as well as any vested interest in a study, such as if a drug or device is being tested that might later be profitable. Questions to ask about conflicts of interest include:

- Was the study externally funded? If so, by whom?
- Are there any potential conflicts of interest?

Activity 6.1　Undertaking a research report critique

1　Search one of your library's databases for a study related to vital signs monitoring in nursing or midwifery, or another topic of personal interest.
2　Work through each of the steps described in this chapter for critiquing published research.
3　Summarise your key conclusions.

Research Example 6.1　Vital signs trends and clinical deterioration

Early recognition of patient deterioration can reduce the risk of potential harm. Timeliness, accuracy and monitoring vital signs trends can be key to early recognition. Brekke et al. conducted a systematic review to evaluate the ability of trends in vital signs to predict clinical deterioration in hospital patients with acute illness. From 7,366 screened references, only two met inclusion criteria but did suggest trend analysis of intermittent vital signs monitoring could increase detection of clinical deterioration. The researchers concluded that there was no consensus on best approaches to analysing trends. They recommended a need for clinical trials with good controls to better understand the value of trends monitoring.

Brekke, I.J., Puntervoll, L.H., Pedersen, P.B., Kellett, J. & Brabrand, M., 2019, 'The value of vital sign trends in predicting and monitoring clinical deterioration: A systematic review', *PLOS ONE*, vol. *14*, no. *1*, e0210875.

Questions for consideration

- How might the findings from systematic reviews be used to support improved practice?
- What does this systematic review indicate about the available knowledge in this field?
- How could Alice in our case study utilise the findings of this review?

Research Example 6.2   A survey to assess nursing students' vital signs monitoring

Recognition of early deterioration is an important role for nurses. Alshehry et al. (2021) conducted a study with 529 undergraduate nursing students to explore perceived knowledge, competence and attitudes towards vital signs monitoring for recognising patient deterioration during clinical placements. The researchers used a survey that covered participant characteristics, education on vital signs in the previous six months, knowledge and competence and a 16-item scale covering key indicators, knowledge, communication, and technology. Findings indicated that students' attitudes were poor, particularly on use of technology in vital signs monitoring, workload associated with vital signs monitoring and vital signs as key indicators of patient deterioration. They concluded there was a need to increase curriculum focus on vital signs monitoring and physiological indicators of clinical deterioration.

Alshehry, A.S., Cruz, J.P., Bashtawi, M.A., Almutairi, K.O. & Tumala, R.B., 2021, 'Nursing students' knowledge, competence and attitudes towards vital signs monitoring during clinical practice', *Journal of Clinical Nursing*, vol. 30, pp. 664–675.

Questions for consideration

- How might the findings from this study inform the delivery of undergraduate education?
- How might the findings of this study assist Alice in our case study in understanding issues in the ward?

Critiquing tools

There are several tools available to assist users of research, as well as researchers, with quality reviews of research studies and working through the increasing amount of research generated. The EQUATOR (Enhancing the Quality and Transparency of Health Research) Network serves as a repository for many critical appraisal tools which have been validated as checklists for different types of research. Examples of these are presented in Research Tip 6.2. In addition, the Joanna Briggs Institute (2023) and the Critical Appraisal Skills Programme (2018; or CASP) have developed suites of critical appraisal tools for a vast array of study designs. Cooper et al. (2021) also produced a set of guidelines for reporting scoping reviews. In addition to their application in assessing study quality, these tools can also be helpful for structuring the writing up of research findings.

Research Tip 6.2   Examples of study reporting guidelines

All are accessible through the EQUATOR Network, at <www.equator-network.org>.

AGREE	Clinical practice guidelines
CARE	Case reports
CONSORT	Randomised controlled trials
PRISMA	Systematic reviews
PRISMA-ScR	Scoping reviews
SQUIRE	Quality improvement studies
SRQR	Qualitative research
STROBE	Observational studies

Activity 6.2   Using critical appraisal tools

1 Using the research article you sourced in Activity 6.1, go to the EQUATOR Network website, at <www.equator-network.org>, the Joanna Briggs Institute website <https://jbi.global/critical-appraisal-tools> and the Critical Appraisal Skills Programme website <https://casp-uk.net/casp-tools-checklists/> and source the appropriate reporting guidelines for the study.
2 Use the reporting guidelines to undertake an evaluation of the quality of the research. Note down your conclusions about the study's quality.

Questions for consideration

- How do your conclusions compare with the review you conducted in Activity 6.1?
- How useful did you find the critical appraisal tools?
- How could the reporting quality of your chosen study be improved?

Structured critical literature review

In the previous part of this chapter, we explored critiquing individual research studies in detail, as well as using critical appraisal tools. In this section, we will look at approaches to performing structured critical reviews of a body of similar work. This is an important practice, as conclusions drawn from such reviews can ensure that the best evidence is applied to nursing and midwifery practice.

Previously, it was acceptable to perform **traditional narrative reviews** of literature. These have no particular approach or structure, are subjective in nature and are often based upon the author's selective approach. Hence, they can be heavily biased and unsystematic (Silva et al., 2022), lack critical appraisal and fail to include the best available research studies. It could be detrimental to base nursing or midwifery practice on the findings of such reviews. Hence, there is a need for very structured, protocol-driven approaches to examining and synthesising the vast amount of literature that may exist on a particular topic in order to extract the best evidence to inform the delivery of care. Among the most common structured critical literature reviews used in nursing and midwifery are the *systematic review* and the *scoping review*.

Systematic review

In this section, we will build on the concept of the **systematic review** introduced in Chapter 1. As its title implies, this type of review is conducted in a systematic way. Systematic reviews have key characteristics and approaches, that include:

• clearly articulated objectives and questions to be addressed
• inclusion and exclusion criteria, outlined in the review protocol/proposal, that determine the eligibility of studies
• comprehensive search to identify all relevant studies, both published and unpublished
• quality appraisal of included studies, assessment of the validity of study results and reporting of any exclusions based on quality
• analysis of data extracted from included research
• presentation and synthesis of findings extracted
• clear and transparent recording of the methodology and methods used to conduct the review.

Systematic reviews provide high-level evidence that can be applied to practice through the synthesis of multiple studies. This synthesis adds strength that may not be achieved through a sole study (Silva et al., 2022).

Developing a review question and PICO

The first step in conducting a systematic review involves developing the research question. This should be carefully thought through, as it needs to be searchable and answerable. It also must incorporate a PICO statement. *PICO* is an acronym used to define the key aspects of a systematic review:

• Population – the types of participants who will be the focus of the review
• Intervention – the intervention or phenomenon of interest that is being examined
• Comparator – what the intervention or phenomenon of interest is being compared with
• Outcome the – outcome measures that are being studied.

There are some variations on the PICO acronym. For systematic reviews of qualitative studies, PICO refers to the following:

• Population – the types of participants who will be the focus of the review
• Phenomenon of interest – the concept being studied
• Context – the setting in which the study should be situated.

Others use *PICOT*, where the *T* refers to a *timeframe*; or *PICOS*, where the *S* refers to *study designs*.

    In this chapter's case study, we could pose the review question: What is the effect of respiratory-rate monitoring in early detection of patient deterioration? For this, our PICO would be:

• Population – deteriorating patients
• Intervention – respiratory-rate monitoring
• Comparator – no respiratory rate monitoring
• Outcome – early detection of deterioration.

Developing the review protocol

Once the question and PICO have been determined, the next step involves developing the **review protocol,** which will direct the search for relevant articles and how these will be analysed and reported. A key part of the protocol involves defining the review's inclusion criteria, which decide whether a study will be included or not and might involve such things as the languages that studies are written in, the timeframe in which research was published, specific characteristics of participants (such as age range or gender), databases and other sources to be searched and the types of studies. The protocol should also identify the quality appraisal tools to be used and how the data will be extracted and analysed.

The review protocol will also include the key search terms (keywords). As we saw in Chapter 2, these can be difficult to determine, need to be constructed in such a way that they will find relevant articles and may vary between databases. Usually, a preliminary list of keywords is developed, followed by detailed development of search strings for each database to be used (see Silva et al., 2022; US National Library of Medicine, 2023). Librarians are highly skilled in formulating search strategies, so seeking their assistance with the formulation of key search terms is advisable. Using our case study, we might develop our protocol in the following way:

- **Inclusion criteria** Quantitative studies published between 2007 and 2017 in English
- **Search strategy**

  - Databases MEDLINE, CINAHL, PubMed
  - Grey literature Google Scholar, professional organisation websites
  - Handsearching Reference lists of retrieved studies
  - Initial key search terms *Patient AND deteriorat* AND nurse AND respiratory rate AND monitor* OR measur* AND detect* AND early OR missed OR late*

- **Quality appraisal** Critical Appraisal Skills Programme checklists appropriate to the studies.

Note the way in which the key terms are shortened when there might be different forms of the same stem word, such as deteriorate, deteriorating and deterioration. By using a truncator symbol (in this case an asterisk), we can find all of these and not miss relevant papers. Note also the reference to grey literature: other relevant studies that might not be listed in databases but might be available from other places—for example, websites of professional or government organisations. You might even use *handsearching*, by looking at reference lists of research studies located in the search to find other studies that may have been missed.

Activity 6.3   Developing a systematic review protocol

Think back to our case study of Alice who was interested in the effectiveness of vital signs monitoring for early detection of patient deterioration. Prior to doing research in her ward, Alice decides to undertake a systematic review of existing literature to explore the topic. She comes up with the following question to guide her systematic review: *How effective are vital signs measurements in detecting early patient deterioration?*

Draft a brief protocol that Alice could use to undertake a systematic review. Use the following headings:

Title
Review question
Background
Inclusion criteria
Participants
Phenomenon or intervention of interest
Outcomes
Study types
Search strategy

Conducting the search, selecting retrieved studies

Once the review protocol has been sufficiently refined, the search is conducted. It is important to keep accurate records of each step. From the initial search, it is common to source large numbers of papers. When numerous databases are being used, first, duplicate records are removed. Following this, the remaining titles and abstracts are read to determine if they fit the inclusion criteria, with those deemed not relevant removed. Ideally, this significantly reduces the number of records. Full texts of the reports that are left are then assessed for inclusion, and again some are normally taken out. This leaves a much smaller number of studies for inclusion in the final review. Often, these steps are presented in a visual Preferred Reporting Items for Systematic Reviews and Meta-Analyses (or PRISMA) flow chart (see <http://prisma-statement.org>). In our case study, the flow chart might look like the one in Figure 6.1.

Appraising retrieved studies, extracting and synthesising data

The quality appraisal tools listed in the review protocol are used to assess the articles included so far. These enable assessment of the quality of the studies included in the final review. At this point, studies not meeting a particular level of quality are removed, and this further reduces the number of studies being included in the final review. According to Porritt et al. (2014), the process of quality appraisal involves establishing risk of bias (in selection, performance, detection and attrition) as well as external validity—how generalisable findings are and, as a result, how applicable they are to making practice changes.

Data extraction and synthesis methods vary; however, protocol development often leads to decisions over what data are important to extract. Usually, these data are presented in the form of tables, which are then interpreted. From this, conclusions can be drawn. At this point, Silva et al. (2022) suggest reporting on the implications for practice according to Joanna Briggs Institute recommendations or similar guideline.

Figure 6.1 Flow chart of a search.

Activity 6.4 Exploring systematic reviews

Using your library's databases, conduct a search for systematic reviews on a topic of personal interest. Identify two or three to read and get a feel for how systematic reviews are reported and presented.

Questions for consideration

- What structure is used to present the findings?
- How are the reviews used to elicit key findings and recommendations that could be translated to practice?

Research Example 6.3   A nursing systematic review

Failure to recognise early change in a patient's status may lead to unnecessary morbidity and mortality. However, how nurses identify changes is unclear. Burdeu et al. (2021) performed a systematic review to examine clinical cues that acute care nurses used to recognise changes in acute patients. They searched across four databases and included 38 studies in the final analysis. The most commonly identified cues were heart rate, blood pressure and temperature. The researchers found studies tended to focus on one particular part of assessment and objective measures. They concluded there was a paucity of studies focusing on the complexity of nurses' assessment practices and identification of patient deterioration.

Burdeu, G., Lowe, G., Rasmussen, B. & Considine, J., 2021, 'Clinical cues used by nurses to recognize changes in patients' clinical states: A systematic review', *Nursing & Health Sciences*, vol. 23, pp. 9–28.

Questions for consideration

- How has the systematic review described above provided greater scope in understanding cues used by nurses in identifying patient deterioration?
- Why is the conclusion from this review more powerful, through combining the findings from a number of research studies, than looking at just one study?

Scoping review

The scoping review is a newer approach to undertaking a structured appraisal of a broad topic of interest and is becoming particularly popular in nursing and midwifery. It reportedly initially emerged in the social sciences, where structured systematic reviews were viewed as very narrow and prescriptive for the types of research conducted in those related disciplines (Thomas et al., 2017). Scoping reviews are applicable to nursing and midwifery, as they incorporate both science and social perspectives. Furthermore, where systematic reviews often focus on the effectiveness of an intervention, scoping reviews seek to expose the gaps in what is currently known about a topic by exploring the breadth of research available on a topic (Munn et al., 2022). This makes them of relevance to the identification of new research opportunities.

While many of the steps undertaken are in line with those of a systematic review, scoping reviews are performed a little differently. They still require the development of a protocol, but rather than using a PICO statement scoping reviews employ different frameworks. The Joanna Briggs Institute approach to scoping reviews suggests a framework encompassing *types of participants, concept* and *context*:

- **Types of participants** This section clearly identifies who the participants of interest are, along with their particular characteristics.
- **Concept** This is the topic being reviewed; it could be an intervention, phenomenon, construct or concept.
- **Context** The context is the specific setting which is being explored—for example, a clinical, community or educational setting (Peters et al., 2020).

Activity 6.5   Developing a scoping review protocol

In our case study, Alice finally decides she needs some more broad information and uses the following question to guide her review: *What is known about nurses' roles in detecting early patient deterioration?*

Draft a protocol for this review, using the following headings, which are informed by the Joanna Briggs Institute (2023) methodology for scoping reviews:

Title
Review question
Background
Inclusion criteria
Types of participants
Concept
Context
Search strategy
Data extraction

Activity 6.6   Exploring scoping reviews

Using your library's databases, conduct a search for scoping reviews on a topic of personal interest. Identify two or three to read and get a feel for how scoping reviews are reported and presented.

Questions for consideration

• What are the key aspects that seem similar across the reviews?
• Are there differences in the ways in which each is presented?
• Are there differences between these scoping reviews and what you have found previously in systematic reviews?

Research Example 6.4   Review of intermittent auscultation in labour

Intermittent auscultation of the fetal heart during labour is usual midwifery practice in managing low-risk women, involving listening to and counting fetal heart rate. Noting little scientific evidence to guide best practice, Blix et al. (2019) undertook a review to identify and synthesise evidence on methods used to perform intermittent auscultation in labour, their effects and accuracy. Searching several databases, they identified 26 studies and 11 guidelines for meta-analysis. Included evidence was evaluated using the GRADE approach. Doppler and Pinard devices were identified as methods used, and abnormal fetal heart rates were detected more with the Doppler. There were no identified differences in neonatal or maternal outcomes, nor any trials recommending the best approach to intermittent auscultation. Overall, the researchers were unable to provide recommendations on a preferred method.

Blix, E., Maude, R., Hals, E., Kisa, E., Karlsen, E., Nohr, E.A., de Jonge, A., Lindgren, H., Downe, S., Reinar, L.M., Foureur, M., Pay, A.S.D. & Kaasen, A., 2019, 'Intermittent auscultation fetal monitoring during labour: A systematic scoping review to identify methods, effects and accuracy. *PlosONE*, vol. *14*, no. *7*, e0219573.

Questions for consideration

- Why was a review the most appropriate approach to address the researchers' questions?
- What can be taken from the review to apply in practice?
- What other evidence might be needed to enable practice recommendations?

Think back to our case study of Alice who was interested in the effectiveness of vital signs monitoring for early detection of patient deterioration. Alice decides she needs to undertake a scoping review to see what is known about nurses' routines in vital signs monitoring. She comes up with the following question to guide her scoping review: What is known about nurses' routines in vital signs monitoring? The question is much broader than it would be for a systematic review. For this, the inclusion criteria would be:

- **Types of participants** – Nurses
- **Concept** – Routines
- **Context** – Vital signs monitoring.

Emerging approaches to literature review

While scoping and systematic reviews are common in nursing and midwifery, there are other types of review emerging in the professions. There are two in particular that can be particularly useful, being rapid reviews and umbrella reviews.

Rapid reviews

Rapid reviews have been widely used in medicine to provide 'actionable and relevant evidence in a timely and cost-effective manner' (Tricco et al., 2017, p. xiii). Thus, they enable fast dissemination and implementation of research into practice, or often, to guide health policy formulation and implementation (Tricco et al., 2017). Recognising that scoping and systematic reviews can take a long time to produce, rapid reviews follow similar review protocols but have more limited inclusion criteria. For example, studies might be included from a smaller publication window or fewer databases might be used.

Umbrella reviews

Umbrella reviews have emerged in nursing and midwifery over recent years. These reviews are usually conducted on topics where there is an abundance of research evidence

---

Activity 6.7   Rapid and umbrella reviews

Search one of your preferred databases for a rapid review and an umbrella review in your discipline area. Consider how the review methods are similar and different to those of systematic and scoping reviews. How might these types of reviews be beneficial to your area of interest?

---

by systematically reviewing and synthesising evidence from multiple systematic and/or scoping reviews. In doing so, they enable the synthesis of large amounts of research evidence with the potential for achieving the highest quality of evidence (Papatheodorou, 2019).

Chapter summary

Evidence to support nursing, midwifery and health professional practice more broadly is flourishing. Nurses and midwives need to possess skills to enable them to sift through the available evidence and effectively critique it for potential implementation into practice and delivery of care. Without such capabilities, patient care may be compromised through implementation of inappropriate or poorly developed research evidence. This chapter has examined processes for critiquing individual research studies and has introduced systematic and scoping reviews as means of collating and critiquing research evidence.

Chapter review questions

- What is meant by *critique* of a research study?
- What are the key aspects to be reviewed in a critique?
- How can author and journal quality be evaluated?
- How are systematic and scoping reviews different?
- Why are systematic and scoping reviews particularly useful in nursing and midwifery?
- What potential do newer types of reviews offer for nursing and midwifery?

Questions for discussion

- How does critiquing research papers challenge traditional narrative literature reviews?
- How might structured critical reviews enhance nursing and midwifery practice?
- What role do traditional narrative literature reviews play?

Questions for personal reflection

- How has your learning from this chapter impacted on your perceptions of doing literature reviews?
- How might it change how you do these in future?
- How might you utilise scoping and systematic reviews in your practice?

Useful web resources

Cochrane <www.cochrane.org>.
Critical Appraisal Skills Programme <www.casp-uk.net>.
Directory of Open Access Journals <https://doaj.org>.
Enhancing the Quality and Transparency of Health Research Network <www.equator-network.
org>.
International Academy of Nursing Editors' Directory of Nursing Journals <https://nursingeditors.
com/journals-directory/>.
International Scientific Institute's Journal Impact Factor List <www.scijournal.org>.
Joanna Briggs Institute <http://joannabriggs.org>.
Preferred Reporting Items for Systematic Reviews and Meta-Analyses <http://prisma-statement.
org>.
SCImago Journal & Country Rank <www.scimagojr.com>.

References and further reading

Alshehry, A.S., Cruz, J.P., Bashtawi, M.A., Almutairi, K.O. & Tumala, R.B., 2021, 'Nursing students' knowledge, competence and attitudes towards vital signs monitoring during clinical practice', *Journal of Clinical Nursing*, vol. *30*, pp. 664–675.

Aromataris, E. & Munn, Z. (eds), 2020, 'JBI Manual for Evidence Synthesis. JBI', <https://synthesismanual.jbi.global>. doi: 10.46658/JBIMES-20-01.

Blix, E., Maude, R., Hals, E., Kisa, E., Karlsen, E., Nohr, E.A., de Jonge, A., Lindgren, H., Downe, S., Reinar, L.M., Foureur, M., Pay, A.S.D. & Kaasen, A., 2019, 'Intermittent auscultation fetal monitoring during labour: A systematic scoping review to identify methods, effects and accuracy', *PLOS ONE*, vol. *14*, no. 7, e0219573.

Brekke, I.J., Puntervoll, L.H., Pedersen, P.B., Kellett, J. & Brabrand, M., 2019, 'The value of vital sign trends in predicting and monitoring clinical deterioration: A systematic review', *PLOS ONE*, vol. *14*, no. *1*, e0210875.

Buccheri, R.K., 2017, 'Critical appraisal tools and reporting guidelines for evidence-based practice', *Worldviews of Evidence-Based Nursing*, vol. *14*, no. 6, pp. 463–472.

Burdeu, G., Lowe, G., Rasmussen, B. & Considine, J., 2021, 'Clinical cues used by nurses to recognize changes in patients' clinical states: A systematic review', *Nursing & Health Sciences*, vol. *23*, pp. 9–28.

Cooper, S., Cant, R., Kelly, M., Levett-Jones, T., McKenna, L., Seaton. P. & Bogossian, F., 2021, 'An evidence-based checklist for improving scoping review quality', *Clinical Nursing Research*, vol. *30*, no. 3, pp. 230–240.

Critical Appraisal Skills Programme, 2018, *CASP Checklists*, <https://casp-uk.net/casp-tools-checklists/>.

Darbyshire, P., McKenna, L., Lee, S.F. & East, C.E., 2017, 'Taking a stand against predatory publishers', *Journal of Advanced Nursing*, vol. *73*, no. 7, pp. 1535–1537.

Joanna Briggs Institute, 2023, *Critical Appraisal Tools*, <https://jbi.global/critical-appraisal-tools>.

McKenna, L., Cooper, S., Cant, R. & Bogossian, F., 2017, 'Research publication performance of Australian professors of nursing & midwifery', *Journal of Advanced Nursing*, doi: 10.1111/jan.13338.

Munn, Z., Pollock, D., Khalil, H., Alexander, L., McInerney, P., Godfrey, C.M., Peters, M. & Tricco, A.C., 2022, 'What are scoping reviews? Providing a formal definition of scoping reviews as a type of evidence synthesis', *JBI Evidence Synthesis*, vol. *20*, no. *4*, pp. 950–952.

Oermann, M.H., Wrigley, J., Nicoll. L.H., Ledbetter, L.S., Carter-Templeton, H. & Edie, A.H., 2020, 'Integrity of databases for literature searches in nursing: Avoiding predatory journals', *Advances in Nursing Science*, vol. *44*, no. 2, pp. 102–110.

Papatheodorou, S., 2019, 'Umbrella reviews: What they are and why we need them', *European Journal of Epidemiology*, vol. *34*, pp. 543–546.

Peters. M., Godfrey, C., McInerney, P., Munn, Z., Tricco, A. & Khalil, H., 2020, 'Chapter 11: Scoping reviews', in E. Aromataris & Z. Munn (eds), *JBI Manual for Evidence Synthesis* [internet], Adelaide: JBI, <https://jbi-global-wiki.refined.site/space/MANUAL>.

Popenoe, R., Langius-Eklöf, A., Stenwall, E. & Jervaeus, A., 2021, 'A practical guide to data analysis in general literature reviews', *Nordic Journal of Nursing Research*, vol. 41, no. 4, pp. 175–186.

Porritt, K., Gomersall, J., & Lockwood, C., 2014, 'JBI's systematic reviews: Study selection and critical appraisal', *American Journal of Nursing*, vol. 114, no. 6, pp. 47–52.

Silva, A.R., Padilha, M.I., Petry, S., Silva, V.S.E., Woo, K., Galica, J., Wilson, R. & Luctkar-Flude, M., 2022, 'Reviews of literature in nursing research: Methodological considerations and defining characteristics', *Advances in Nursing Science*, vol. 45, no. 3, pp. 197–208.

Thomas, A., Lubarsky, S., Durning, S.J. & Young, M.E., 2017, 'Knowledge synthesis in medical education: Demystifying scoping reviews', *Academic Medicine*, vol. 92, no. 2, pp. 161–166.

Tricco, A.C., Langlois, E.V. & Straus, S.E. (eds), 2017, *Rapid Reviews to Strengthen Health Policy and Systems: A Practical Guide*, Geneva: World Health Organization. Licence: CC BY-NC-SA 3.0 IGO.

US National Library of Medicine, 2023, *Medical Subject Headings*, <www.nlm.nih.gov/mesh/>.

7 Ethics and research in nursing and midwifery

Learning objectives

After working through this chapter, you should be able to:

- Discuss the role of Human Research Ethics Committees (HRECs)
- Describe the principles underpinning the ethical conduct of research
- Identify researchers' responsibilities in ensuring their research is ethical
- Identify bodies responsible for formulating policy in research ethics
- Discuss issues relating to using web-based and social media sources for research

Key terms and concepts

Approval processes, beneficence/non-maleficence, ethical principles, ethics, Human Research Ethics Committees, justice, research integrity, research merit, respect for persons.

Case study overview

Michael is the nurse unit manager in a busy medical ward. Current ward policy is that all patients have their vital signs recorded every four hours, regardless of their condition. He feels this is inefficient in terms of making best use of nursing staff's time, that it does not promote critical-thinking skills and that it is ineffective in detecting patient deterioration. He suggests that individualising frequency of vital signs measurement according to patient condition would be more effective. He proposes to undertake a randomised controlled trial comparing current practice with individualised practice to determine whether nurses' abilities to detect patient deterioration improve.

Chapter introduction

It is vital that researchers protect the rights of the people they study. In health research in particular, the people who are the subjects, or the participants, of research are often in a state of vulnerability. Rules or guidelines to ensure that research is conducted ethically, and that participants' rights are protected are a relatively recent development. In this chapter, we will examine the governance of human research ethics, including the approval and monitoring processes. We will discuss the principles of ethical research conduct and procedures by which researchers can ensure they are followed.

DOI: 10.4324/9781003414476-10

Development of ethical principles in research

The question of ethics in research gained widespread attention after the Second World War when the experiments conducted by Nazi doctors in concentration camps came to light. However, there have been many other instances where research participants have not been treated ethically, both before and since. The first guideline on the ethical conduct of research was produced in 1947, following the verdict in the so-called Doctors' Trial at Nuremberg, Germany, and is thus known as the Nuremberg Code (Shuster, 1997). The code established ten principles for properly designed scientific studies involving humans and the treatment of research participants.

Building on this, in 1964, the World Medical Association (2013) produced its version of ethical research principles, in the Declaration of Helsinki, based on a framework of universal human rights. It was addressed primarily to physicians undertaking medical research, but anyone conducting research into people's health was encouraged to abide by it. The declaration is an evolving document, taking into account developments in medicine and health care and the need for more complex research. It has been amended several times. It is internationally accepted and forms the basis for all national guidelines.

In many countries, the ethical conduct of research is governed by one or more central bodies, such as the Australian National Health and Medical Research Council (NHMRC), the Health Research Council (HRC) and the National Ethics Advisory Committee in New Zealand, the Health Research Authority in England (in collaboration with devolved administrations in Scotland, Wales and Northern Ireland), and the Office for Human Research Protections (OHRP) in the USA. The OHRP (2022) has compiled a list of standards for human research from 131 countries and many international organisations. All researchers conducting research with people are expected to have read the standards relevant to the country in which they are doing the research, and to abide by the principles, as are bodies responsible for approving and monitoring research studies.

Human Research Ethics Committees

The oversight of the ethical conduct of research involving people is the responsibility of bodies variously called Research Ethics Committees, Human Research Ethics Committees (HRECs), Institutional Ethics Committees and Institutional Review Boards. (The word *human*, when used, is included to distinguish the process from animal research, which has slightly different guiding principles and processes.) This text will refer to them as HRECs for clarity and simplicity. HRECs are established in hospitals, universities and several other institutions. They are usually convened and regulated by national or regional governing bodies (Health Research Authority, 2021; HRC, 2012; NHMRC, 2007/2023). The requirements for the composition of an HREC vary but typically include a mix of professional and lay people, a mix of genders and people with sufficient expertise to be able to evaluate proposals on a range of topics; it is common for a lawyer to be included, and ethical expertise may be required. In New Zealand, at least one person must have awareness and understanding of Māori culture (HRC, 2012).

The role of HRECs is to ensure that research undertaken within their institutions, or by people affiliated with them (usually employees, but also students in the case of universities), complies with ethical standards. They review research proposals and grant or deny approval for the research to be undertaken. They are also responsible for monitoring

---

Activity 7.1   Human Research Ethics Committees

1 Locate information about the HREC responsible for approving research in your institution.
2 Obtain the application form and read the questions, relating them to the principles of ethical conduct described below: *research merit and integrity, beneficence and non-maleficence, respect for persons* and *justice*.

Questions for consideration

• What are the procedures necessary for applying for ethical approval in your institution?
• What forms need to be completed?
• Are there different levels of approval for different types of research?
• Are all the ethical conduct principles listed above covered in the application form?
• Are there any questions on the form that do not relate to the principles?

---

studies that have been approved, usually through annual reports submitted by researchers, though additional processes may be required in cases of high-risk research.

It should be noted that decisions about the ethics of conducting research are not always straightforward, and different HRECs do not always reach the same decisions. Ethical standards are not a set of rules to be followed mechanically. As the Australian NHMRC states, application of the guidelines 'always requires, from each individual, deliberation on the values and principles, exercise of judgement, and an appreciation of context' (NHMRC, 2007/2023, p. 11).

Principles of ethical conduct of research

Ethical conduct of research continues to be underpinned by a framework of universal human rights. While the rights of participants in research are the primary concern, the rights of the wider community and of researchers themselves are also taken into account. There are four universally accepted principles of ethical conduct: *research merit and integrity, beneficence and non-maleficence, respect for persons* and *justice*.

Research merit and integrity

This principle is underpinned by the belief that research must be free from major flaws and carried out honestly. It should be obvious that research fraud and misconduct are unethical (even illegal in some cases); it may be less obvious that poor quality research can also have ethical implications. The rationale is that practice based on evidence that is unreliable, for whatever reason, is potentially dangerous (Moore et al., 2010).

The concept of research merit precludes research being undertaken for no good reason. It requires that there is potential benefit from any research; depending on the topic and the procedures involved, this could simply mean contributing to a body of knowledge.

Researchers are required to provide full justification for their proposed research, including showing how it fits with what is already known (through a literature review). It is not ethical to continue researching a procedure or therapy if there is already strong evidence for or against its use. A component of research merit is ensuring that the research question can be answered and the potential benefit realised. This includes demonstrating that the design is appropriate to answer the question, that the sample size is appropriate (too small and the question may not be answered; too large and participants could be exposed to unnecessary risks), that the researchers have sufficient experience and qualifications to undertake the research and that necessary facilities and resources are available. All these factors should be demonstrated in the research proposal.

Research integrity means that research must be conducted and reported honestly. A consensus statement on research misconduct in the UK (2012) listed the following types of misconduct:

> fabrication [of data or of entire studies]; falsification, suppression, or inappropriate manipulation of data; inappropriate image manipulation; plagiarism; misleading reporting; redundant publication; authorship malpractice such as guest or ghost authorship; failure to disclose funding sources or competing interests; misreporting of funder involvement.

Other examples include manipulating study procedures to make it more likely that a desired outcome is achieved, and selective reporting of outcomes (Moore et al., 2010). Unfortunately, research misconduct, whether deliberate or unintentional, appears to be a growing problem (Boetto et al., 2021); it is estimated that it makes up nearly 20% of medical literature (Cogan, 2022).

A number of codes of conduct are available to assist researchers in good research practice and to avoid misconduct. Codes have been developed within countries, such as in Australia (NHMRC, 2018a) and the UK (UKRIO, 2023) and across countries, such as the European code (ALLEA, 2023). The codes set out responsibilities of both institutions and researchers and emphasise the need for study procedures to be transparent and auditable and therefore carefully documented. Standards for recording and managing data to minimise the possibility of fraud are included. Training and mentoring of junior researchers are also addressed. The codes mention standards for disseminating research findings, which have been further developed by the international Committee on Publication Ethics (or COPE). The standards include requirements for authors to declare any conflicts of interest and standards on what constitutes authorship (preventing 'honorary' authorship and making all named authors responsible for the content of a paper).

Boetto et al. (2021) call for journal policies to be tightened to reduce the incidence of flawed research, either through falsification or serious error, being published. The extent of the problem in nursing and midwifery research is unknown (Gray, 2018). Al-Ghareeb et al. (2018) conducted a systematic review to examine the rates at which papers in nursing and midwifery journals were retracted (removed). They found that rates were low compared with other disciplines, but that retracted studies continued to be cited. Further analysis found that 23 systematic reviews included retracted papers as part of the study, suggesting that flawed research may be influencing nursing and midwifery practice (Gray et al., 2018).

Beneficence and non-maleficence

The principle of beneficence and non-maleficence is underpinned by the belief that people have the right not to be harmed. The requirement is that the likely benefits of research must outweigh any risk of harm or discomfort. The benefits may be to the participants themselves, to the wider community or to both. This principle is not just concerned with physical harm; participants can suffer emotional, psychological, financial, social or legal harm, depending on the purpose of the research. Researchers are responsible for assessing the known risks and designing research to minimise them. This could mean testing procedures beforehand to ensure their safety or taking steps to prevent harm. For example, financial harm may result if participants incur expenses as part of their role in the research; this can be avoided by reimbursing them for any expenditure. Any risks must be made known to potential participants. Researchers are also responsible for ensuring the welfare of participants during (and possibly after) the research. Procedures for managing potential risks and reporting any unintended outcomes must be built into the research proposal.

In assessing risk, researchers and ethics committees have to take into account both the severity and the likelihood of the risk. *Severity* can be classified under the levels harm, discomfort and inconvenience:

- **Harm** Can range from extreme, such as major morbidity or even death, to relatively minor, such as temporary distress from reliving unpleasant experiences in an interview or experiencing unpleasant side-effects of medications.
- **Discomfort** Less serious than harm; it can be physical or emotional and may result from very minor side-effects of medications or stress from taking part in an interview or being observed at work, for example.
- **Inconvenience** Less serious again; it can occur with activities such as filling in a form or taking time to participate in research.

Likelihood is the possibility of adverse outcomes occurring. For example, there may be a very remote chance (say, 1 in 10,000) of major physical harm resulting from the study procedures. While this should not be discounted, it will most probably not be counted as a major risk. The possibility of discomfort could be very high (close to 100%), and while this would probably be counted an acceptable risk, the researchers would still need a plan to manage it. Studies can be classed as *low risk* if the only likely adverse outcome is discomfort and as *negligible risk* if the only foreseeable risk is inconvenience. Ethics committees often have different procedures for each risk level.

In this chapter's case study, the outcome in Michael's proposed trial is patient deterioration, either detected by nurses and managed appropriately or not detected, with the consequent risk of a poor outcome for the patient. This constitutes harm. Even though this is a risk with current practice, it will be considered in assessing the risk of the study. Michael will have to argue that the study carries sufficient likely benefit to outweigh the potential for harm. Although he hopes that the new practice will reduce the number of patients whose deterioration is not detected, he does not know that it will do so (otherwise, there would be no point in doing the research), and there is a possibility that the opposite will happen: that the number will be increased. Because the severity of harm is high, Michael will need a plan for monitoring patient welfare during the study.

Activity 7.2   Risks of research

The following case studies were discussed in Chapters 4 and 5.

1   Marek plans a quasi-experimental study to see if a nurse education program can improve person-centred care. He plans to measure person-centred care before and after the program to see if there is a difference. Two potential studies are suggested:

- Person-centred care is measured by surveying patients to determine their satisfaction with care.
- Person-centred care is measured by surveying nurses to determine the extent to which it is practised.

2   Stephanie proposes to measure person-centred care in her ward to determine how well it is practised. Two ways of doing this are suggested:

- Nurses are observed in their practice, with the number of times they practise in a person-centred way noted.
- Nurses are surveyed with the same tool as that used by Marek.

3   Jill plans to interview nurses on her ward to explore their understanding of person-centred care.

Questions for consideration

- What risks do you consider there are to participants in each of these scenarios?
- How might the researchers manage the risks?
- Are there any risks to the researchers?

While risks to participants are the main concern of those overseeing research, in some situations the researchers themselves may be at risk as well. Physical harm can result from research procedures. Research carried out in the workplace is subject to usual health and safety regulations and should therefore require no additional precautions. However, if research is conducted outside the workplace—for instance, in field work or by going into participants' homes—a risk assessment for the researcher should be made and a plan put in place (Butler et al., 2019). Researchers can also be at risk of psychological or emotional harm if researching a sensitive topic; of social harm if, for example, their relationships are affected; and of academic or professional harm if their research findings are controversial.

Respect for persons

This principle is underpinned by the belief that people have a right to self-determination. The principle is sometimes referred to as autonomy but is actually broader than this. The basic concept is of informed consent: that research should not be carried out on people without their knowledge and permission. This is a legal as well as an ethical imperative. Note that there is no such thing as uninformed consent—no one can be deemed to consent to something of which they have no knowledge or understanding.

Ensuring that participants are informed requires researchers to provide full disclosure on what is involved in taking part in the research, including any risks that may be involved, as well as the consequences of not taking part. This latter point is very important when testing or evaluating new practices, such as new therapies; patients need to know what care they will receive if they decline to be in the study. A minimum requirement is that information be provided in writing, in a document called a *participant information statement*. Information must be provided in a language and at a level that people can readily understand. Researchers must make every effort to overcome any other factors that may limit people's ability to understand the material. For example, people in a highly stressful situation—such as sudden illness—are less likely to be able to assimilate information. Researchers can help by providing time for people to consider whether they want to take part and opportunities for them to ask questions about the research.

When they have sufficient information to make an informed decision, potential participants are asked to provide their consent to take part in the research. Consent can be provided in a number of ways. In most research in which the researchers and participants have direct contact, written—signed—consent is required. This is the equivalent of signing a legal document. Occasionally, verbal consent may be sufficient; this is likely to occur in low-risk situations. Sometimes, consent can be implied by the participant's continuing with the study procedures. The commonest scenario of **implied consent** is that of a survey, where filling out and returning or submitting a questionnaire can be interpreted as the person's consenting to take part in the study.

In some studies, it can be difficult or even impossible to obtain informed consent at the time that potential participants need to be enrolled. Examples include emergency situations involving unconscious patients, and women in the second stage of labour. Sometimes, seeking formal consent can impose an unnecessary risk or burden on participants. Several alternative methods for obtaining consent have been developed to enable research to be undertaken in these situations. One is **deferred** or **retrospective consent**. This method was used in a study to evaluate myocardial injury in critically ill patients in Intensive Care Units; data collection required collection of blood samples and electrocardiograms over a period of time (Honarmand et al., 2018). At the time data collection had to commence, many patients were too ill to provide consent. Eligible patients were therefore enrolled without consent, then, later, either they or their next of kin were told about the study and asked if they wanted to remain in it. If they did not, they were removed from the study and their data deleted. Another alternative is the opt out method. This is most often used in relation to routinely collected health data, which may be used later for research purposes, or studies which have minimal impact on participants. An example is a study to test and refine a tool to enhance decision-making about admission or discharge of children in Emergency Departments (Long et al., 2022). Parents were told about the study, and that their child's routinely collected data would be used in the study unless they chose not to participate. In other circumstances, the need to obtain consent can be waived altogether, although this is quite controversial.

Specific guidelines have been developed for the protection of populations deemed to be vulnerable, including those who are unable to provide consent for themselves. This category includes people who are unconscious, people who are mentally impaired, and children, all of whom are protected by legislation determining who can consent on their behalf. Pregnant women and fetuses are also numbered among the vulnerable populations, as are some ethnic minorities. In Australia, there are specific guidelines for research involving Aboriginal and Torres Strait Islander peoples (NHMRC, 2018b), while New Zealand standards (2022) specifically require researchers to consider the impact of their research on Māori and Pacific Islander peoples.

Another important point about consent is that it must be freely given; that is, people must not be coerced into taking part. The information given to potential participants must always include a statement to the effect that participation is voluntary and that declining to participate will not result in any adverse effects—for example, patients' medical care will not be affected in any way. However, this statement may be insufficient: people may still feel pressured to take part. This is particularly the case if there is an unequal relationship between researchers and potential participants or if researchers are in a position of authority over potential participants. Examples of unequal relationships include health professionals and patients in their direct care, employers and employees, managers and subordinates, and teachers and students.

Also underpinning this principle is people's right to privacy. **Privacy** is enshrined in legislation, as well as being an ethical requirement. These laws may operate at national level or in smaller jurisdictions; in Australia, for instance, every state and territory has its own privacy legislation. Researchers need to be aware of, and comply with, the relevant laws. They include ensuring that data are securely stored both during and after a study, so that unauthorised persons do not have access to them; not revealing information that participants want kept confidential; and usually not revealing in reports any information that could identify the participants. The last of these requirements can extend to institutions—for example, not revealing the name of a hospital where the research was carried out. The most complete protection of identity is conferred by anonymity, in which the researchers do not know who the participants are. This is possible in many surveys but rarely in other types of research. It should be noted that if researchers promise participants that they will be anonymous, written consent—which requires people's names to be recorded—cannot be requested. This is the reason that implied consent is acceptable in this situation.

Activity 7.3   Informed consent

In our case study, patients in Michael's ward are an ethnically diverse group, and many have limited English-language skills. Moreover, a large proportion of patients have low literacy and numeracy skills.

Questions for consideration

- What challenges do these factors present in gaining informed consent?
- What strategies could Michael use to ensure consent is truly informed?

Activity 7.4   Clinical relationships

In the case study in Chapter 5, Jill, the unit manager on a busy medical-surgical unit, plans to undertake a qualitative study with the nurses in her ward, because she is concerned that the nursing care is not person centred; that is, she perceives there is a deficit in the care being given.

Questions for consideration

- What ethical concerns might be raised by the relationship between Jill and her staff?
- What strategies could Jill employ to overcome these concerns?
- Is there a possibility of an unequal relationship in the research?

Justice

The principle of justice is underpinned by the belief that people have a right to be treated fairly. It requires that the following conditions are met:

- Recruitment procedures are fair. This includes taking steps to ensure that anyone who might benefit from taking part in the study has the opportunity to do so. One reason for the requirement for registration of clinical trials is to enable people to search the registry to find out if there are any studies relevant to them.
- Participants are not exploited.
- Study procedures are fair to all participants and do not place an undue burden on any specific group. For example, if some people are required to travel long distances to take part in a study, they might either decide not to take part (thus missing out on any potential benefit), or they might take part but then be disadvantaged financially.
- Any benefits of participating in research are fairly distributed.
- Access to benefits of research findings is fair.
- Research outcomes are made available to all participants.

Reporting on ethical practices

To be considered by a reputable journal, manuscripts reporting on research studies must demonstrate that the study has been approved by the relevant HREC(s), and usually researchers are required to provide the approval number. Beyond this, there is little to no consistency in what details are provided. If the processes undertaken by researchers are not described, readers cannot judge whether the research was conducted ethically (McKenna & Gray, 2018). It is important, therefore, for practices relating to all the ethical principles to be described in as much detail as necessary for this judgement to be made. This is the responsibility of journal editors and peer reviewers, as well as researchers.

Activity 7.5   Exploring research ethics

Find a research report on any topic of interest to you.

Questions for consideration

- What information is included in the report about ethical issues? For example, is approval mentioned? Do the authors indicate how they addressed ethical concerns? Do they mention consent?
- Can you identify any ethical issues that are not mentioned?
- Do you consider that the authors have addressed ethical issues and their management in sufficient detail? If not, what other details would you like to have seen?

Research Example 7.1   Ethical issues in collecting data by observation

Monitoring vital signs is an important component of nursing practice and ensuring patient safety. It is a practice performed frequently so that any deterioration in a patient's condition can be detected early, but the impact on nursing workload is unclear; this makes it difficult to plan staffing appropriately. Dall'Ora et al. (2021) conducted a study to determine how much times nurses spend measuring and recording patients' vital signs, and to identify factors that influenced the amount of time.

The study was conducted in 16 adult general medical and surgical wards in four public hospitals in the UK. All nursing staff working on the ward at the time of each observation session were asked to participate. Two researchers observed nurses' practice during 64 separate sessions and recorded the start and stop times, and any interruptions that occurred. They also recorded the number of patients on the ward and the number and levels of nursing staff. After the session, they asked the nurses if their behaviour had changed as a result of being watched. The researchers observed 715 sets of vital signs measurement, of which 680 were deemed complete. They also recorded 1,695 interruptions, 496 of which were related to the actual taking of vital signs (such as replacing faulty equipment). They found that monitoring and recording a single set of vital signs took an average of 3.75 minutes spent at the bedside. The researchers concluded that the workload in monitoring vital signs is considerable and that any change in the frequency of monitoring has implications for resource allocation.

Dall'Ora, C., Griffiths, P., Hope, J., Briggs, J., Jeremy, J., Gerry, S. & Redfern, O.C., 2021, 'How long do nursing staff take to measure and record patients' vital signs observations in hospital? A time-and-motion study', *International Journal of Nursing Studies*, vol. *118*, p. 103921. doi: 10.1016/j.ijnurstu.2021.103921.

Questions for consideration

- What ethical issues could be of concern in this study design?
- How would these issues be addressed to ensure the ethical conduct of research and patient safety, bearing in mind that the patients were not the study participants?

Research Example 7.2   Ethical issues in collecting data by survey

Physical assessment of patients is an essential nursing role to detect changes in a patient's condition in a timely manner. Rosli et al. (2023) conducted a study to determine what, and how frequently, physical assessment was undertaken by critical care nurses in Malaysia, and what factors influenced this. The study was conducted in three critical care units in one hospital. Potential participants, based on the inclusion criteria, were identified by the head nurse. Study packages, consisting of an envelope containing a questionnaire labelled with an individual identification number, a study information sheet and consent form, were distributed to 140 nurses in the units. Participants were asked to complete the questionnaire within seven days and return it to the nursing supervisor. A member of the research team visited the site once a week to collect the completed surveys. The survey tool included demographic data, 40 questions regarding how often physical assessment techniques were performed, and open-ended questions about issues that nurses perceived influenced the skills they used. From 133 completed questionnaires, the researchers found that nurses with more experience performed assessment more often than those with less, but all scored poorly in areas such as auscultation. Participants indicated that more continuing education and standardised assessment reporting would enhance their practice.

Rosli, S.N., Soh, K.L., Ong, S.L., Halain, A.A., Abdul Raman, R. & Soh, K.G., 2023, 'Physical assessment skills practised by critical care nurses: A cross-sectional study', *Nursing in Critical Care*, vol. *28*, no. *1*, pp. 109–119. doi: 10.1111/nicc.12748.

Questions for consideration

- What are the ethical issues in this study?
- What procedures should the researchers follow to ensure compliance with all the principles of ethical research conduct?

Internet and social media use in nursing and midwifery research

Many health professionals, including nurses and midwives, seek to use the internet and social media to access data for research. While it may be tempting to engage in collecting data from such sources, due to the ready availability of extensive pools of data, Lunnay et al. (2015) suggest that researchers need to be clear about the benefits of approaching social media for research activity. From an ethical perspective, having readily available research data raises a number of issues, and HRECs are increasingly having to consider applications proposing to use such sources. One issue is that data are potentially identifiable; for example, if taken from Facebook posts, data could be linked back to a person whose identity may be revealed. Also, people usually post to social media sites for personal reasons but not for the purpose of their posts being used for research purposes. Hence, they probably have not provided consent for the use of their posts, even though they are in the public domain.

Activity 7.6   Using social media sources in research

Think about your own social media use.

Questions for consideration

- Is there content that you post that could be used as research data?
- How might you feel if you were to see your posts directly used in research studies?
- What could be the potential benefits of using internet and social media content as data sources, particularly in nursing and midwifery research?

Chapter summary

Protection of both research participants and researchers is fundamental to good research practice. Ethical standards for conducting research have been established internationally and are governed locally. These standards are based on four guiding principles: research merit and integrity, beneficence and non-maleficence, respect for persons and justice. In this chapter, processes for the approval and monitoring of ethical conduct of research have been discussed. Finally, the area of ethical issues surrounding research using the internet or social media sources has been explored.

Chapter review questions

- What institutions are responsible for providing guidance and advice on ethical conduct of research in the UK and Australia?
- What is the role of HRECs?
- What is meant by each of the following:

  - research merit and integrity
  - beneficence and non-maleficence
  - respect for persons
  - justice?

- What procedures can researchers follow to ensure ethical principles are upheld?
- What ethical issues may arise in research using the internet or social media as data sources?

Questions for discussion

- Why is ethics so important for research in health care?
- How can you determine whether research evidence has been generated ethically?
- What are the implications for nursing and midwifery if research is not ethical?
- How could we effectively use the internet or social media for meaningful nursing and midwifery research?

Questions for personal reflection

- What have you learnt from this chapter about best practice in conducting research ethically?
- How will this impact on your reading of research reports?

Useful web resources

Committee on Publication Ethics <https://publicationethics.org>.
Health Research Authority UK <https://www.hra.nhs.uk/about-us/>.
Health Research Council of New Zealand <https://www.hrc.govt.nz/>.
National Health and Medical Research Council on Ethical Issues <www.nhmrc.gov.au/health-ethics/ethical-issues-and-further-resources>.
UK Research Integrity Office <https://ukrio.org/>.

References and further reading

A consensus statement on research misconduct in the UK, 2012. BMJ; 344: e1111

Al-Ghareeb, A., Hillel, S., McKenna, L., Cleary, M., Visentin, D., Jones, M., Bressington, D. & Gray, R., 2018, 'Retraction of publications in nursing and midwifery research: A systematic review', *International Journal of Nursing Studies*, vol. *81*, pp. 8–13. doi: 10.1016/j.ijnurstu.2018.01.013.

ALLEA, 2023, *The European Code of Conduct for Research Integrity – Revised Edition 2023*, Berlin. doi: 10.26356/ECOC.

Boetto, E., Golinelli, D., Carullo, G. & Fantini, M.P., 2021, 'Frauds in scientific research and how to possibly overcome them', *Journal of Medical Ethics*, vol. *47*, p. e19.

Butler, A., Copnell, B. & Hall, H., 2019, 'Researching people who are bereaved: Managing risks to participants and researchers', *Nursing Ethics*, vol. *26*, no. *1*, pp. 224–234. doi: 10.1177/0969733017695656.

Cogan E. Preventing fraud in biomedical research. Front Cardiovasc Med. 2022, vol. *9*, 932138. doi: 10.3389/fcvm.2022.932138.

Dall'Ora, C., Griffiths, P., Hope, J., Briggs, J., Jeremy, J., Gerry, S. & Redfern, O.C., 2021, 'How long do nursing staff take to measure and record patients' vital signs observations in hospital? A time-and-motion study', *International Journal of Nursing Studies*, vol. *118*, p. 103921. doi: 10.1016/j.ijnurstu.2021.103921.

Doody, O. & Noonan, M., 2016, 'Nursing research ethics, guidance and application in practice', *British Journal of Nursing*, vol. *25*, no. *14*, pp. 803–807.

Gray, R., 2018, 'Why are so few nursing science papers retracted?', *Nurse Author and Editor*, vol. *28*, no. *3*, pp. 1–7.

Gray, R., Al-Ghareeb, A., Davis, J., McKenna, L. & Hillel, S.S.A., 2018, 'Inclusion of nursing trials in systematic reviews after they have been retracted: Does it happen and what should we do?', *International Journal of Nursing Studies*, vol. *79*, p. 154.

Health Research Authority, 2021, *Governance Arrangements for Research Ethics Committees*, <https://s3.eu-west-2.amazonaws.com/www.hra.nhs.uk/media/documents/GAfREC_Final_v2.1_July_2021_Final.pdf>.

Health Research Council of New Zealand (HRC), 2012, *Guidelines for Approval of Ethics Committees*, <http://www.hrc.govt.nz/sites/default/files/2019-06/Resource%20Library%20PDF%20-%20Approval%20guidelines%20November%202012.pdf>.

Honarmand, K., Belley-Cote, E.P., Ulic, D., Khalifa, A., Gibson, A., McClure, G., Savija, N., Alshamsi, F., D'Aragon, F., Rochwerg, B., Duan, E.H., Karachi, T., Lamontagne, F., Devereaux, P.J., Whitlock, R.P. & Cook, D.J., 2018, 'The deferred consent model in a prospective observational study evaluating myocardial injury in the intensive care unit', *Journal of Intensive Care Medicine*, vol. *33*, no. *8*, pp. 475–480. doi: 10.1177/0885066616680772.

Im, E.O. & Chee, W., 2012, 'Practical guidelines for qualitative research using online forums', *CIN: Computers, Informatics, Nursing*, vol. *30*, no. *11*, pp. 604–611. doi: 10.1097/NXN.0b013e318266cade.

Ingham-Broomfield, R., 2017, 'A nurses' guide to ethical considerations and the process for ethical approval of nursing research', *Australian Journal of Advanced Nursing*, vol. *35*, no. *1*, pp. 40–47.

Long, T., Rowland, A., Cotterill, S., Woby, S., Heal, C., Garratt, N., Brown, S. & Roland, D., 2022, 'Opt-out consent in children's emergency medicine research', *Comprehensive Child and Adolescent Nursing*, vol. *45*, no. *1*, pp. 31–42. doi: 10.1080/24694193.2020.1812766.

Lunnay, B., Borlagdan, J., McNaughton, D. & Ward, P., 2015, 'Ethical use of social media to facilitate qualitative research', *Qualitative Health Research*, vol. *25*, no. *1*, pp. 99–109.

Mahon, P.Y., 2014, 'Internet research and ethics: Transformative issues in nursing education research', *Journal of Professional Nursing*, vol. *30*, pp. 124–129.

McKenna, L. & Gray, R., 2018, 'The importance of ethics in research publications', *Collegian*, vol. *25*, no. *2*, pp. 147–148.

Moore, R.A., Derry, S. & McQuay, H.J., 2010, 'Fraud or flawed: Adverse impact of fabricated or poor quality research', *Anaesthesia*, vol. *65*, no. *4*, pp. 327–330. doi: 10.1111/j.1365-2044.2010.06295.x.

New Zealand National Ethical Standards, 2022, National Ethics Advisory Committee (NEAC), <https://neac.health.govt.nz/national-ethical-standards/>.

NHMRC, 2007, *National Statement on Ethical Conduct in Human Research*, updated 2023, Canberra: Commonwealth of Australia.

NHMRC, 2018b, *Ethical Conduct in Research with Aboriginal and Torres Strait Islander Peoples and Communities: Guidelines for Researchers and Stakeholders*, Canberra: Commonwealth of Australia.

NHMRC, Australian Research Council & Universities Australia, 2018a, *Australian Code for the Responsible Conduct of Research*, Canberra: Commonwealth of Australia.

Office for Human Research Protections (OHRP), 2022, International Compilation of Human Research Standards, <https://www.hhs.gov/ohrp/international/compilation-human-research-standards/index.html>.

Rosli, S.N., Soh, K.L., Ong, S.L., Halain, A.A., Abdul Raman, R. & Soh, K.G., 2023, 'Physical assessment skills practised by critical care nurses: A cross-sectional study', *Nursing in Critical Care*, vol. *28*, no. *1*, pp. 109–119. doi: 10.1111/nicc.12748.

Shuster, E., 1997, 'Fifty years later: The significance of the Nuremberg Code', *New England Journal of Medicine*, vol. *337*, pp. 1436–1440.

UK Research Integrity Office, 2023, *Code of Practice for Research*, <https://ukrio.org/wp-content/uploads/UKRIO-Code-of-Practice-for-Research.pdf>.

World Medical Association, 2013, *Declaration of Helsinki: Ethical Principles for Medical Research Involving Human Subjects*, <www.wma.net/policies-post/wma-declaration-of-helsinki-ethical-principles-for-medical-research-involving-human-subjects/>.

Zimmer, M. & Kinder-Kurlanda, K., 2017, *Internet Research Ethics for the Social Age: New Challenges, Cases, and Contexts*, New York: Peter Lang.

Section 4

How Do I Use Evidence to Inform My Practice?

The previous sections in this book have explored the nature of evidence in nursing and midwifery, where and how to source it and make sense of it. In this section, we take the next step, exploring how evidence can be applied to nursing and midwifery to make a difference to our care of people. Knowledge translation—the translation of research-based evidence into practice—is imperative if that evidence is to make a real difference.

Chapter 8 specifically explores the processes by which knowledge can be translated into practice. It explores how nurses and midwives can question their practice to enhance the care they deliver.

An important skill for nurses and midwives is the writing of literature reviews. In Chapter 6, we introduced the systematic and scoping reviews as examples. Chapter 9 examines the writing of literature reviews, which you may be required to produce as a student or for colleagues in clinical practice, and how to approach it.

Once new knowledge is generated through reviews or research, it is important for these to be shared, or disseminated, so others may be able to utilise it. Chapter 10 explores ways by which outcomes can be disseminated through professional presentations and publication.

DOI: 10.4324/9781003414476-11

8 Applying evidence in practice

Learning objectives

After working through this chapter, you should be able to:

- Discuss the importance of evidence-based practice (EBP) in nursing and midwifery
- Identify who is responsible for the translation of knowledge to practice
- Outline the role of clinical practice guidelines and clinical audit in EBP
- Discuss some of the models that can be used to guide evidence implementation
- Discuss ways to evaluate the implementation of new evidence into practice
- Identify factors impacting on the implementation of evidence into practice

Key terms and concepts

Action research, evidence implementation, implementation science, knowledge translation, realist evaluation.

Case study overview

John is a clinical nurse specialist on a busy medical-surgical ward. He is concerned about a recent rise in medication errors in the ward. He decides to examine the available evidence in the area and explore the current practices in the ward to see if they are impacting on the rising error rates.

Chapter introduction

Evidence-based practice (EBP) is an important part of nursing and midwifery. Research is growing rapidly; however, much of the evidence generated may never be translated into practice. Just as research needs to be conducted systematically and thoroughly, so too does the translation of new knowledge into clinical practice. This requires a process for implementing the evidence, as well as for evaluating its effectiveness at the local level. In this chapter, we will explore the process for doing that, through the concept of **knowledge translation**, models and processes for implementing evidence into practice and strategies for evaluating its impact.

DOI: 10.4324/9781003414476-12

Responsibility for knowledge translation

One of the challenges facing researchers and clinicians is the divide between the generation and the implementation into practice of research knowledge. Whose responsibility is the implementation of new knowledge into clinical practice? The only people who can realistically be responsible for this are clinicians, regardless of their area of practice. They are providing the care and as such, have the contact with the people receiving the care informed by the research. That being said, researchers have a responsibility to be doing the types of research that clinicians need to inform their practice. As we highlighted in Chapter 1, various countries' standards require nurses and midwives to use evidence to support their care, reinforcing their roles and responsibilities in this regard. In addition, some professional organisations, such as the Australian Nursing and Midwifery Federation, have developed their own policies for research and EBP.

It is widely recognised that it is not appropriate for decisions about care delivery to be based upon what has been traditionally done or to be made according to the preference of the care provider. Rather, care decisions need to be driven by the best available research evidence. While this sounds logical, many challenges have been faced by nurses and midwives in applying EBP and hence in the delivery of best-practice care (Leach & Tucker, 2018).

Activity 8.1   Responsibility for knowledge translation

In this chapter's case study, John is concerned about the rising medication error rate on his ward.

Questions for consideration

- Who in the ward is responsible for the review of new evidence regarding medication administration practices?
- What factors have influenced your views on this allocation of responsibility for evidence application?

Activity 8.2   Reflecting on knowledge translation

Think of a clinical practice area where you have recent experience.

Questions for consideration

- Was knowledge translation considered to be important?
- Whose role was specifically related to knowledge translation?
- Who else had some responsibility for knowledge translation in that area?
- From where was new knowledge sourced to inform practice change?
- Did you observe a clinical audit or use of clinical practice guidelines informing practice?

Questioning clinical practice

In order to recognise a need for new evidence to support practice, it is necessary to question the existing practice. It is not sufficient to continue traditional practice just because it has always been done that way. It may not be delivering the best practice to those people who are receiving care. It is essential to constantly question clinical practice. Some questions that can be asked are:

- What is the current practice?
- Why is it undertaken that way?
- What evidence is it based upon?
- Is newer evidence available?
- Is a change in practice feasible in this clinical setting?

However, questioning clinical practice can be challenging, particularly in areas where the same staff have been working and delivering care together in the same ways for many years. Implementing practice change cannot be effectively undertaken by one person; rather, a team-based approach is crucial to implementing and maintaining any new practice. Garnering support for change will be important for ensuring its relevance to practice and the potential for successful implementation.

Sources of evidence for practice

We have closely examined the role of research literature in informing EBP. However, there are other sources from which credible knowledge to inform clinical practice can be drawn, as described below.

Clinical practice guidelines

These are guidelines for clinical practice that have been developed based on the best available evidence, so a lot of the work around sourcing and evaluating evidence has already been conducted. **Clinical practice guidelines** allow healthcare professionals to make sound decisions and deliver optimal care in specific circumstances. Organisations, such as hospitals, often develop clinical practice guidelines specifically in their own settings. In Australia, the National Health and Medical Research Council developed Standards for Guidelines (2016) to assist with development and implementation and has a searchable repository for guidelines. New guidelines are assessed according to the Standards, considering their value to decision-making, transparency, process for development, evidence-informed, actionable and current (NHMRC, 2016). In the United Kingdom, the National Institute for Health and Care Excellence (or NICE) has an extensive bank of clinical practice guidelines and audits <www.nice.org.uk> and contains a large number of clinical practice guidelines specific to nursing.

Clinical audit

Clinical audits are commonly used in health care to measure aspects of performance. They form an important aspect of clinical governance and quality improvement and can be conducted at ward or organisation level. Limb et al. (2017) present clinical audit as a cyclical process with six stages, as reproduced in the list below, to which we have added brief explanations:

1 **Identifying a problem** Initially identifying the problem and local resources needed for the audit.
2 **Defining standards/criteria** deciding what is to be measured and the performance standard desired
3 **Collect data** collecting data to enable evaluation of the problem and current performance
4 **Analysis** analysing the data and comparing it with the desired level of performance
5 **Implementing change** implementing necessary change to achieve desired target
6 **Re-audit** monitoring (including potential repeat audits) and sustaining change (Limb et al., 2017).

Implementing evidence into practice

The implementation of new evidence into clinical practice requires a team-based, structured approach. Tucker and Melnyk (2019) define 12 steps that provide a logical way to approach implementation of evidence into practice. These include:

1 Use sound data and rationale to identify whether and why a change in practice is needed.
2 Assess readiness for change in the organisation, along with its strengths and potential barriers.
3 Create a vision for change that is communicated to all staff and key stakeholders.
4 Source input on the vision from key stakeholders.
5 Convene teams of key stakeholders to develop a plan with goals that are **SMART** (specific, measurable, action-focused, realistic, time-sensitive).
6 Provide preparation, tools and resources for leaders.
7 Leverage relevant networks, champions, and mentors.
8 Utilise evidence-based implementation approaches to promote and sustain change.
9 Harness small changes to encourage and motivate ongoing changes.
10 Regularly recognise and appreciate participation and progress.
11 Monitor progress and modify plans as needed.
12 Share progress and outcomes with stakeholders and celebrate achievement of goals.
(Tucker & Melnyk, 2019, pp. 6–9)

Activity 8.3 Questioning clinical practice

Think about a clinical skill that you are familiar with and how you have seen that skill performed in practice. Use the questions at the beginning of this section to conduct an evaluation of the skill as you saw it in practice.

Questions for consideration

- Was that practice based on best available evidence?
- How might a clinical audit be employed to improve it?

Evidence-based practice models

Numerous models have been developed and employed by nurses and midwives to facilitate the successful application of evidence to their practice. In this section, we will take a look at a selection of these models.

Activity 8.4   Evidence implementation

In our case study, John is concerned about the rising medication error rate on his ward. He uses a questioning approach to consider the current medication administration practice in the ward, discovering that many practices are not evidence based. He decides to review clinical practice guidelines and to undertake a clinical audit. From these, he confirms that current medication management practices are not evidence based or ensuring the delivery of optimal quality care. He sets about forming a team to work on implementing new EBP.

Questions for consideration

- What skills might be needed in the team?
- Who might be key people in the team?
- What else needs consideration?
- What should John do once he has the team together?

Research Example 8.1   Examining evidence-based nursing and midwifery practice

EBP combines best available evidence, health professionals' expertise and patient preference, and it can be challenging to implement. In the Republic of Ireland, Cleary-Holdforth et al. (2021) used a survey approach to explore nursing and midwifery clinicians', educators' and students' beliefs, knowledge and implementation of EBP. All groups displayed positive beliefs about EBP, but their abilities to do this and actual implementation were low. The groups held varying perceptions of organisational support and readiness for EBP. Clinicians identified insufficient mentors or champions, financial support, decision-making capability and commitment to EBP. Educators and students identified having computer proficiency and access to electronic databases as strengths. Students also identified having academics who were EBP champions as another strength.

Cleary-Holdforth, J., O'Mathuna, D. & Fineout-Overholt, E., 2021, 'Evidence-based practice beliefs, implementation, and organizational culture and readiness for EBP among nurses, midwives, educators, and students in the Republic of Ireland', *Worldviews on Evidence-Based Nursing*, vol. 18, no. 6, pp. 379–388.

Questions for consideration

* Do you think the findings of this study might be similar elsewhere, that is, transferable?
* How might these findings be used to inform the development of EBP?

Johns Hopkins Nursing Evidence-Based Practice Model

The Johns Hopkins Nursing Evidence-Based Practice Model for Nursing and Healthcare Professionals provides a structured decision-making approach to applying evidence to clinical nursing practice. It uses a three-step process referred to as *PET: practice question and project planning, evidence* and *translation*. Within the model are 20 steps to guide EBP. Various tools are provided to guide teams through the process, from development of the initial question to dissemination of findings arising from the process (Johns Hopkins Health System/Johns Hopkins School of Nursing, 2022).

Promoting Action on Research Implementation in Health Services

In 1998, Kitson et al. developed the Promoting Action on Research Implementation in Health Services (or PARIHS) framework. This approach to knowledge translation is underpinned by the concept that 'successful implementation of research in practice is a function of the relation between the nature of the evidence, the context in which the proposed change is to be implemented and the mechanisms by which the change is facilitated' (Kitson et al., 1998, p. 150). The authors introduced the formula:

$$SI = f(E, C, F)$$

where successful implementation (SI) is a function (f) of evidence (E), context (C) and facilitation (F). In the model, there is an emphasis on the facilitator, who works with people to see the need for change and in making the change happen. It has been widely implemented across a range of implementation projects (Bergström et al., 2020).

Advancing Research and Clinical Practice through Close Collaboration

The Advancing Research and Clinical Practice through Close Collaboration (or ARCC©) model takes a very different, behavioural approach to effective implementation of evidence into practice, being underpinned by control theory and cognitive behavioural theory. It comprises an initial assessment at organisational level of existing EBP culture and readiness, and identification of strengths and potential barriers. It has, at its core, the development and use of mentors in EBP to promote its implementation with a view to improving patient outcomes, staff satisfaction and reducing costs to health services (Melnyk et al., 2017).

Activity 8.5   Exploring an evidence-based practice model

1 Select an EBP model, either from those above or another you are aware of.
2 Search for some literature where that model has been utilised.
3 Summarise how the model was used in evidence implementation.

Questions for consideration

- How successful was the implementation?
- Were there any challenges reported by the authors in applying the model?

Evaluation of practice change

Across the 2000s, we saw the evolution of **implementation science,** a science focused on implementing evidence for practice change. Westerlund et al. (2019, p. 332) suggest 'the ambition to generate knowledge to promote a better uptake of evidence for improvements in the quality and safety of health care' emerged due to a distinct gap between research and its application. However, the implementation of new evidence is not complete just with practice change. It is important to know if the change makes a difference and whether it is appropriate. One of the limitations regularly stated in research papers is that the findings may not be generalisable to any other population beyond that included in the study. Whenever new evidence is being implemented, there may be differences in the practice setting that influence its usefulness. Hence, evaluation of the implementation of new knowledge is vital to ensure it makes a positive change. Such evaluation can form a type of research study in its own right—hence, again, the need for nurses and midwives to possess some research knowledge and skills. Evaluation might constitute a range of data collection tools, such as questionnaires, interviews and observations. There are numerous approaches to evaluating evidence implementation. In this section, we will look at two approaches, *participatory action research* (PAR) and *realist evaluation*, which both develop and implement new evidence for practice.

Participatory action research

PAR is a practical research approach that has been used for many years in nursing and midwifery, among other disciplines. The *action* nature of this approach makes it unique in practice change. It is known as a *participatory* approach to research, because the participants are actively involved as members of the research team, helping to guide its progress as well as to allow participants to be empowered. According to Schubotz (2019), PAR enables researchers 'to utilise the research process in order to change and improve the situations of those being researched'.

PAR occurs in a cyclical process with participants as research team members, hence values the experience and knowledge they bring. There are four steps involved in this approach that may be repeated many times as the research unfolds. In each step, there may be different elements of data generated, depending on what is being explored:

1 **Define the problem** The first step is defining the problem to be addressed, developing common understandings and planning the action to be taken.
2 **Action** The plan from the previous step is implemented. In the case of a practice change, it is in this stage that the new practice is trialled as the group has previously determined.
3 **Observation** Implementation of the plan is monitored and collaboratively assessed. This includes deciding whether there are changes required or other issues arising that need to be considered.
4 **Reflection** The plan is reflected on, reviewing its implementation and any other considerations, redesigning actions and plans for the next cycle.

The number of cycles in action research studies will vary across projects. However, generally, they have a timeframe determined by the research team (Cornish et al., 2023).

Research Example 8.2   Participatory action research in implementation of evidence-based practice

PAR is often applied in nursing and midwifery to facilitate practice change. In Australia, Radbron et al. (2022) used PAR to explore how nurses and midwives used patient experience data to influence person-centred practice across six clinical units in one health district. They used three action cycles to collect data via a mobile application on staff perceptions of person-centredness, as well as conducting 17 interviews. Over the project, the researchers noted improved person-centredness among staff along with changes to culture and practice through use of the application.

Radbron, E., Wilson, V., McCance, T. & Middleton, R., 2022, 'The experience of staff utilizing data to evaluate and improve person-centred practice: An action research study', *Journal of Advanced Nursing*, vol. 78, pp. 3457–3469.

Questions for consideration

• Why was action research an appropriate choice for this study?
• Why was it a more appropriate approach than another such as phenomenology or grounded theory?
• How can findings from action research, such as this, lead to enhanced care delivery?
• What might be the benefits of using action research in nursing and midwifery practice settings?

Activity 8.6   Participatory action research

Think about your current area of practice. Can you identify a clinical practice that could be changed using a PAR approach? How might you go about such a project?

Questions for consideration

- What aspects of the practice need to change?
- What is the context in which the research will occur?
- Who will need to be involved?
- How many cycles might be needed? What will these entail?

Data collection in participatory action research

During the process of PAR, a range of data can be collected. Their purpose is to provide evidence to support the practice change. Data can be quantitative (such as questionnaires, experimental studies and auditing of clinical documentation) or qualitative (interviews, observations and focus groups) in nature, or both, and often various approaches are employed. All will aid in evaluating the effectiveness or impact of the practice change.

It would be easy to conduct an implementation process and call it an action research study. However, as with any research study, action research needs to be conducted in a rigorous and defendable way. Effendy et al. (2022) conducted a scoping review to explore implementation of PAR in nursing. Twenty studies were included in the review that utilised elements of PAR. They found around 65% of studies used principles of participation in study design, with around 35% using collaborative design through meetings and dialogue and 70% used participants in data collection. Only 25% described participatory dissemination of findings. They concluded that elements of PAR were being used by nurses but highlighted the need for benefits to be reciprocated for researchers and participants (Effendy et al., 2022).

Realist evaluation

Realist evaluation is an increasingly popular approach, particularly in health care, to examine the nature of programs and how they work, for the purpose of refining or testing theory. It translates research approaches into the domains of policy and practice that stresses the importance of stakeholders in the process. The methodology varies but can employ qualitative or quantitative methods, depending on the evaluation (Pawson & Tilley, 1997, 2004).

The process of realist evaluation involves four main concepts, as outlined by Pawson and Tilley (2004); we have once again added explanations to their list:

1 **Mechanism** the nature of programs or interventions that actually bring about effects
2 **Context** the context in which programs are introduced or delivered
3 **Outcome patterns** the outcomes of the program, both intended and unintended
4 **Context mechanism outcome pattern configuration** the way in which all concepts work together overall; also called CMOC.

Realist evaluation, like action research, is conducted in a four-stage research cycle. Our explanations follow the stages as listed by Pawson and Tilley:

1 **Hypothesis** Information is accessed and theory formulated about what in the program 'works for whom in what circumstances'.
2 **Data collection** Data are collected on the mechanisms, contexts and outcomes of the program and can be diverse, with information drawn from such sources as question-naires, interviews and observations.
3 **Data analysis** Data are analysed to explore outcome patterns and examine which of these can be explained through the initial theory and which cannot.
4 **Theory testing** Understandings of the context mechanism outcome pattern configuration are revised and it is decided if another cycle is needed (Pawson & Tilley, 2004, p. 24).

Activity 8.7   Realist evaluation

Think about the clinical practice that you used in Activity 8.6.

Questions for consideration

• Could realist evaluation be used to implement and evaluate the required change?
• If not, why not?

Research Example 8.3   Realist evaluation of nursing practice

In England, Jeffries et al. (2017) conducted a realist evaluation to examine the implementation of a new electronic system for optimising a drug administration system into a general practice context. They conducted five semi-structured in-terviews, four focus groups and one observation with key stakeholders. The re-searchers found that the system improved patient safety outcomes and there was better identification of patients who were at risk of developing adverse drug events. However, they also concluded that effective use depended on how engaged health professionals were with the system and the information flow between the different professionals.

Jeffries, M., Phipps, D.I., Howards, R.L., Avery, A.J., Rodgers, S. & Ashcroft, D.M., 2017, 'Understanding the implementation and adoption of a technological intervention to improve medication safety in primary care: A realist evaluation', *BMC Health Services Research*, vol. 17, article 196.

Questions for consideration

• Why was realist evaluation an appropriate design for this study?
• How might the findings lead to enhanced care delivery?

Research Example 8.4   Realist evaluation of midwifery continuity of care

Midwifery **continuity of care** (CoC) has been a focus for improving the quality of care provided, and perinatal outcomes, for childbearing women. In Scotland, McInnes et al. (2018) used realist evaluation to monitor the implementation of midwifery CoC in one health board area. They developed a framework for evaluating clinical outcomes for women and midwives through the implementation process. They identified the importance of staff involvement and ongoing evaluation to assess progress in successful implementation and sustaining the midwifery CoC model into the future. Furthermore, their tools could potentially be used in other health services seeking to make similar changes.

McInnes, R.J., Hollins Martin, C.J. & MacArthur, J., 2018, 'Midwifery continuity of carer: Developing a realist evaluation framework to evaluate the implementation of strategic change in Scotland', *Midwifery*, vol. 66, pp. 103–110.

Questions for consideration

- Why was realist evaluation an appropriate design for this project?
- How might the outcomes lead to enhanced care delivery?

Chapter summary

Nurses and midwives need to have the knowledge and skills to implement new knowledge into practice, to ensure they deliver best practice. Successful implementation of EBP requires a systematic and well-informed approach. This chapter has introduced the concept of knowledge translation and processes for questioning current practices. It has examined places for sourcing quality evidence, and processes and structures that can be employed to successfully implement new evidence into practice.

Chapter review questions

- Why is implementation of new evidence into nursing and midwifery practice important?
- Who is responsible for implementing new evidence into practice?
- Why is evaluation of implementation of new practice needed?
- How can approaches such as action research and realist evaluation assist with evaluating practice change?

Questions for discussion

- What might be facilitators and barriers to the implementation of new evidence into clinical nursing or midwifery practice?
- What strategies could be used to manage these?

Questions for personal reflection

- How much do you consider evidence in your own practice?
- What might assist you to be more focused on evidence in your practice?

Useful web resources

Australian Nursing and Midwifery Federation's Nursing and Midwifery Research Policy <http://anmf.org.au/documents/policies/P_Nursing_Midwifery_Research.pdf>.

Johns Hopkins Medicine's Johns Hopkins Nursing Evidence-Based Practice Model <www.hopkins-medicine.org/evidence-based-practice/ijhn_2017_ebp.html>.

National Health and Medical Research Council (2016) NHMRC Standards for Guidelines <https://www.nhmrc.gov.au/guidelinesforguidelines/standards>.

National Institute for Health and Care Excellence (United Kingdom) <www.nice.org.uk>.

References and further reading

Bergström, A., Ehrenberg, A., Eldh, A.C., Graham, I.D., Gustafsson, K., Harvey, G., Hunter, S., Kitson, A., Rycroft-Malone, J. & Wallin, L., 2020, 'The use of the PARIHS framework in implementation research and practice: A citation analysis of the literature', *Implementation Science*, vo. *15*, no. *68*.

Casey, M., O'Leary, D. & Coghlan, D., 2017, 'Unpacking action research and implementation science: Implications for nursing', *Journal of Advanced Nursing*, vol. 74, no. 5, pp. 1051–1058.

Cleary-Holdforth, J., O'Mathúna, D. & Fineout-Overholt, E., 2021, 'Evidence-based practice beliefs, implementation, and organizational culture and readiness for EBP among nurses, midwives, educators, and students in the Republic of Ireland', *Worldviews on Evidence-Based Nursing*, vol. *18*, no. 6, pp. 379–388.

Cornish, F., Breton, N., Moreno-Tabarez, U., Delgado, J., Rua, M., Aikins, A.D. & Hodgetts, D., 2023, 'Participatory action research', *Nature Reviews Methods Primers*, vol. *3*, no. *34*.

Effendy, C., Margaretha, S.E.P.M. & Probandari, A., 2022, 'The utility of participatory action research in the nursing field: A scoping review', *Creative Nursing*, vol. *28*, no. *1*, pp. 54–60.

Jeffries, M., Phipps, D.L., Howards, R.L., Avery, A.J., Rodgers, S. & Ashcroft, D.M., 2017, 'Understanding the implementation and adoption of a technological intervention to improve medication safety in primary care: A realist evaluation', *BMC Health Services Research*, vol. *17*, article 196.

Johns Hopkins Health System/Johns Hopkins School of Nursing, 2022, *Johns Hopkins Evidence-Based Practice Model for Nursing and Healthcare Professionals*, <https://www.hopkinsmedicine.org/evidence-based-practice/model-tools.html>.

Kitson, A.L. & Harvey, G., 2016, 'Methods to succeed in effective knowledge translation in clinical practice', *Journal of Nursing Scholarship*, vol. *48*, no. *3*, pp. 294–302.

Kitson, A.L., Harvey, G. & McCormack, B., 1998, 'Enabling the implementation of evidence based practice: A conceptual framework', *Quality in Health Care*, vol. 7, pp. 149–158.

Leach, M.J. & Tucker, B., 2018, 'Current understandings of the research-practice gap in nursing: A mixed-methods study', *Collegian*, vol. *25*, pp. 171–179.

Limb, C., Fowler, A., Gundogan, B., Koshy, K. & Agha, R., 2017, 'How to conduct a clinical audit and quality improvement project', *International Journal of Surgery. Oncology*, vol. 2, no. 6, p. e24.

McInnes, R.J., Hollins Martin, C.J. & MacArthur, J., 2018, 'Midwifery continuity of carer: Developing a realist evaluation framework to evaluate the implementation of strategic change in Scotland', *Midwifery*, vol. 66, pp. 103–110.

Melnyk, B.M., Fineout-Overholt, E., Giggleman, M. & Choy, K. 2017, 'A test of the ARCC© model improves implementation of evidence-based practice, healthcare culture, and patient outcomes', *Worldviews on Evidence-Based Nursing*, vol. 14, no. 1, pp. 5–9.

National Health and Medical Research Council *see NHMRC*

NHMRC, 2017, *Clinical Practice Guidelines Portal*, <www.clinicalguidelines.gov.au/portal>.

Nilson, P., 2015, 'Making sense of implementation theories, models and frameworks', *Implementation Science*. doi: 10.1186/s13012-015-0242-0.

Pawson, R. & Tilley, N., 1997, *Realistic Evaluation*, London: Sage.

Pawson, R. & Tilley, N., 2004, *Realist Evaluation*, Community Matters, <www.communitymatters.com.au/RE_chapter.pdf>.

Radbron, E., Wilson, V., McCance, T. & Middleton, R., 2022, 'The experience of staff utilizing data to evaluate and improve person-centred practice: An action research study', *Journal of Advanced Nursing*, vol. 78, pp. 3457–3469.

Rowles, E. & McNaughton, A., 2017, 'An overview of the evidence-based practice process for novice researchers', *Nursing Standard*, vol. 31, no. 43, pp. 50–60.

Schubotz, D., 2019, 'Participatory Action Research', in P. Atkinson, S. Delamont, A. Cernat, J.W. Sakshaug & R.A. Williams (eds), *SAGE Research Methods Foundations*. doi: 10.4135/9781526421036840298.

Tucker, S. & Melnyk, B.M., 2019, 'A leader's guide to implementing evidence-based practice', *American Nurse Today*, vol. 14, no. 6, pp. 6–9.

Westerlund, A., Nilsen, P. & Sundberg, L., 2019, 'Implementation of implementation science knowledge: The research-practice gap paradox', *Worldviews on Evidence-Based Nursing*, vol. 16, no. 5, pp. 332–334.

9 Writing effective reviews of literature

Learning objectives

After working through this chapter, you should be able to:

- Discuss why literature reviews are important for evidence-based nursing and midwifery practice
- Identify different types of literature reviews
- Outline the key reasons for performing a literature review
- Identify steps involved in developing a quality literature review
- Plan and write a quality literature review

Key terms and concepts

Direct quotation, grey literature, literature review, paraphrasing, primary source, secondary source, synthesis.

Case study overview

April is a first-year student who has been given the following assignment for her clinical subject, in which medication management has just been introduced: 'With reference to the literature, critically explore issues around medication administration by nurses and midwives'. April recognises that to do this, she needs to do a literature review. She has never written a formal review before and does not really know how to go about it.

Chapter introduction

In Chapter 6, we explored different types of literature reviews commonly used in nursing and midwifery—namely, the traditional narrative review, systematic review and scoping review. We also explored the processes for searching for literature and critically appraising it. This chapter builds on that content to examine the process of making sense of the research literature and putting it together in a meaningful and quality review that can form a basis on which to deliver evidence-based practice.

DOI: 10.4324/9781003414476-13

What is a literature review?

A **literature review** is 'a comprehensive overview of literature related to a theme/theory/ method and synthesizes prior studies to strengthen the foundation of knowledge' (Paul & Criado, 2020, p. 1). A sound literature review provides an overview of the key ideas around what is known on the topic of interest. In addition, it identifies where there are gaps in what is known on the topic and where future research might be warranted.

Literature reviews are commonly allocated as academic assessment tasks. However, the skills needed for conducting and writing them are also important for nursing and midwifery practice. Clinical guidelines to inform practice should be developed after rigorous reviews of previous studies have ensured that all appropriate evidence on which to base that practice has been appraised and synthesised. The ability to communicate findings of such a review is also therefore paramount to the development of strong clinical guidelines (Murad, 2017). According to Leite et al. (2019), literature reviews serve a number of purposes, including the following:

- Provide a sound framework of what research has been performed on a topic.
- Identify topics requiring further research.
- Identify previous methodologies and methods used to explore an area.
- Enable assessment on the context or scope of a problem.

Types of literature reviews

There are many types of literature reviews. They can be descriptive or traditional in nature, such as narrative review, purely describing the available literature, or they can take a very structured approach, such as in a systematic or scoping review (Silva et al., 2022). To inform evidence-based practice, preference is given to reviews that have structured search strategies and processes for synthesis and analysis, as well as including quality appraisal of included studies.

Activity 9.1   Types of literature reviews

- Review the types of literature reviews presented in Chapter 6.
- Summarise the key differences between them.

Research Example 9.1   Scoping review of nurse fatigue and medication administration error

Medication administration is a key component of the nurse's role. Errors in medication administration pose major risks to patient safety, so understanding causes of errors is important for practice. Bell et al. (2023) conducted a scoping review of literature to explore the impact of fatigue on medication errors and near misses by hospital registered nurses. They included 38 papers dating from 1992 to 2021 and originating predominantly from Iran and the United States. They analysed how medication administration error was defined, and how it was impacted by fatigue across 31 of the papers. Overall, they identified two themes: *shift work and the effect on sleep cycle,* and *the RNs' hours or work.* Overall, they found that shift schedules, shift length, overtime work, and sleep restriction all played a role. However, they did find large inconsistencies across papers in the degree to which these were factors in medication administration errors. They recommended that larger studies were needed to explain the inconsistencies.

Bell, T., Sprajcer, M., Flenady, T. & Sahay, A., 2023, 'Fatigue in nurses and medication administration errors: A scoping review', *Journal of Clinical Nursing*. doi: 10.1111/jocn.16620.

Questions for consideration

- How could the findings from this scoping review help to guide medication administration practice?
- How could collating research findings from a number of studies like this assist us to better understand the area of medication administration?

Research Example 9.2   Narrative review of medications and breastfeeding

Sometimes medication administration to mothers can lead to early cessation of breastfeeding. McClatchey et al. (2018) undertook a narrative literature review to investigate factors relating to medicine safety that could contribute to medication unnecessarily becoming a barrier to breastfeeding. Using a number of relevant databases, they searched using the search terms *breastfeeding, lactation, medication* and *information*. They then reviewed the 657 articles retrieved, finding 145 were eligible for complete text review. These were evaluated to determine if they identified the need for medication potentially or actually impacting on decision to breastfeed and 40 were included in the final review. From their analysis, the researchers determined that need for medication could influence early breastfeeding cessation. They found the main limitations to sound advice were a lack of available information and inconsistency within evidence-based resources.

McClatchey, A.K., Shield, A., Cheong, L.H., Ferguson, S.L., Cooper, G.M. & Kyle, G.J., 2018, 'Why does the need for medication become a barrier to breastfeeding? A narrative review', *Women and Birth*, vol. 31, pp. 362–366.

Questions for consideration

- How could the findings from this narrative review help to guide midwives' practice?
- How could collating research findings from a number of studies like this assist us to better understand medication administration in midwifery?

Writing a literature review

Clarifying the question

Before embarking on a literature review, it is important to understand what is required of the review. If it is for an academic assignment and the topic is provided, it is crucial to carefully consider what is being asked and what the keywords are in the question. If the topic has to be determined, consider a question that is not too broad and can be easily managed. You can get a sense of how much literature is available on a topic by doing a quick database search. If the topic appears to have been very well researched, narrow the focus to something more manageable. It will be much easier to move on to the detailed search if the question is well crafted beforehand. University and hospital librarians can be of great assistance in helping to refine literature searches, so it may be useful to seek one out at this point.

Searching for literature

In Chapters 2 and 6, we touched on searching for literature and quality appraisal of research. Before you can undertake a review, you need to determine the **keywords** that you are going to use to search for relevant literature. These will be directly related to your research question or topic but you need to consider variations, such as synonyms, for each word to ensure the review is broad enough. To do this effectively takes time, but it will enhance the quality of the review. As identified in Chapter 2, the US National Library of Medicine (2023) has a very useful website of Medical Subject Headings, where you can search for additional keywords and extend the literature search to ensure as many articles as possible are captured.

At this point, it is also important to consider what you will include in your review. It is common practice to decide on a date range from which literature will be sourced. If you are performing a review of research for current practice, it is not sensible to draw recommendations from outdated research. As a rule of thumb, literature should be no more than ten years old. However, for some clinical practices or academic requirements much more recent literature might be required, particularly if the aim is to identify gaps in current knowledge. On the other hand, you may need to go further back than ten years when knowledge is well established and does not need to be researched again. It is important also to decide whether only research studies—quantitative, qualitative or both—will be included in the review or whether other types of materials, such as reports, clinical guidelines and discussion papers, will be included, and why.

Literature for review can be accessed from multiple sources. However, it is necessary to check the quality of the material you source and only use that which you can clearly see is credible. Most resources are likely to come from databases accessed through your university or hospital library. In addition to material sourced through databases, you can also seek out grey literature, for example, reports or clinical guidelines available from other sources, such as professional and government organisations. The search engine Google Scholar can be particularly useful in searching for other types of credible materials that might not be listed on databases.

There are some important tricks in searching for appropriate research literature. One of these is using **truncations**—that is, parts of words that may appear in different forms. This concept was introduced in Chapter 2, so you may wish to review that chapter before you continue on.

Activity 9.2   Searching for literature

In this chapter's case study, first-year student April needs to do a literature review for one of her assessment tasks. She has been asked to use literature to critically explore issues around medication administration by nurses and midwives.

1 Develop a list of keywords that April could use to search for relevant literature.
2 Using these keywords, go to one of the databases in Research Tip 2.1 that you have not used before and conduct a search. Try including some Boolean operators and truncators in the format for that database.
3 List the challenges you encounter.
4 Search on Google Scholar for literature that may assist April.

Questions for consideration

• What differences do you note between the relevance and specificity of hits from the database and the search engine?
• How might these differences impact on the way you use each?

Selecting literature to include

Generally, a search of databases will yield many more articles than you need for a review. However, many may also be irrelevant to the topic you are exploring, or they may not meet your initial inclusion criteria. In Chapter 6, we examined the process of determining the scope of systematic and scoping reviews. Sometimes, these approaches can also be useful in facilitating more focused narrative reviews. In addition, the tools covered in that chapter provide a foundation for determining the quality of the research evidence and could be used to assist with deciding what to include in a more general review.

Reading and critiquing the literature

Careful reading and re-reading of each sourced paper is needed to fully grasp the main concepts presented in it. As you do this, it is important to write in your own words notes of your interpretations of the key aspects. This helps to ensure you have fully understood the paper and the author's discussion. Begin to group papers into those with similar focuses. This will assist you when it comes to planning out the review. Remember to note down the relevant details required for referencing the paper, to make the process of writing the report smoother.

Consider also the nature of the material. Papers that you use in your review should be **primary sources**; that is, the research should be directly reported by the researchers who actually conducted the research study. **Secondary sources** are those where the authors are reporting on someone else's research, so they provide a second-hand account of the work. In this case, they may not give an accurate description of the actual research study. If you notice you have a secondary reference, it is best to seek out the original or to not make use of the work in your review. Textbooks are usually considered secondary references, unless they are providing first-hand reports of research written by the researchers who conducted the study.

Synthesising ideas and planning the review

Just like planning for any essay, a written plan is important for ensuring that a clear line of argument and flow of ideas appears in the final review. This should include an introduction, body and conclusion. For a high-quality review, careful planning of ideas and their flow is needed.

Introduction

The review will begin with an introduction. This establishes and explains the argument that the paper is making, defines any keywords or terminology and provides necessary background to the topic. It gives the reader an idea of the direction that the review will take.

Review body

The body of the literature review provides the main discussion and argument. From your reading and summarising, you will have ascertained the key ideas and concepts to be covered. These will become the topic sentences presenting the key messages that will subsequently form each of the paragraphs. It is important to organise these ideas in such a way that the overall content and argument flow logically from the beginning to the end of the work. Thus, the ideas covered in each paragraph should build on those in the previous paragraph and lead into those in the next.

Conclusion

The conclusion draws together the key ideas presented in the work. It might also include discussion of limitations in the existing body of literature and make recommendations for future research.

Writing the review

Once you have developed the plan for your literature review, you can begin to write. As you do this, you will need to present the ideas from the research papers you have read and summarised. However, the review should not just read like a list of quotations or jump from idea to idea without a clear flow. The reader should be led from a very broad, general introduction of the topic to a specific focus. It needs to be clear that you have synthesised and carefully considered the ideas of different authors and are not just reporting their findings one after the other. Remember that you need to create a consistent line of argument that flows throughout the work. Your plan should have been developed in such a way as to allow you to create meaningful paragraphs that fit together seamlessly. Any claims made or conclusions presented in the review need to be supported by appropriate research evidence.

Paraphrasing is an important strategy in academic writing. This involves rewriting key ideas in your own words. Many people make the mistake of merely replacing a few words throughout a piece of text and believing they have paraphrased. This is not considered to be paraphrasing; rather the material needs to be rewritten in other words but retaining the concept, argument or idea that the original author was making. Whenever you are presenting the ideas of another author or researcher—that is, not your own original thoughts—you must also cite the person (or people) who originally documented them.

Activity 9.3 Paraphrasing

1 Source the full text of one of the research articles on medication administration issues that you located for Activity 9.2.
2 Select one or two paragraphs and paraphrase the key points that the author is making in them.
3 Note down your experiences of doing this.

Question for consideration

• What things did you need to be mindful of?

You can also use **direct quotations** to support arguments—that is, word-for-word text from a research paper. However, it is a good idea to keep these to a minimum where possible, for use when a concept is too difficult to paraphrase or with ideas that are fundamental to the research. Present direct quotations clearly, in quotation marks, indicating that the work is that of another author. Many referencing style approaches, for example, APA or Harvard, will also require you to add the page number of the original source.

The word length of a quotation will determine where in the text it is placed. Depending on the referencing style used, quotes longer than 30 to 40 words may start on a new line and be indented. If your literature review has a prescribed word count, remember that quotations generally do not contribute to it, as they do not constitute your own words.

The way your work will be interpreted by an independent reader needs careful consideration as you write. While you will likely know all the studies covered in your review very well, the reader may not. You need to provide enough detail of each study for the reader to understand the context and the argument that you are making. In our case study, for example, April could write in her review, 'Williams et al. (2023) found that nurses were often distracted during medication administration'. However, the reader would understand much more of the context of the study if April wrote this along the lines of 'Williams et al. (2023) found using observational methods that nurses in two hospitals in Australia were often distracted by other health professionals, patients and telephone calls during medication administration'.

It is important to present a balanced perspective. Not all research that you include will necessarily support your original assumptions. Noting differences in study designs and outcomes, and conflicting findings as well as similar findings, should form part of the picture. Keep in mind that while you may have a particular belief about the topic, very different findings may emerge from the literature. The review should not reflect your personal beliefs; rather, it must reflect what is actually presented through the literature.

Research Example 9.3   Systematic review of double checking to reduce medication errors

Medication administration forms a large part of nursing and midwifery work, and errors pose a major risk to patient safety. Double checking of medications has been a longstanding strategy for reducing errors, but its effectiveness has also been debated. Koyama et al. (2020) conducted a systematic review to explore the evidence around double checking on reducing medication administration errors. They identified 13 articles meeting their inclusion criteria that included ten observational studies, two randomised controlled trials and one randomised trial in a simulation context. Of the included studies, there was 52% to 97% reported adherence with double checking. However, none of the studies examined whether there was a change in error rates due to double checking. The researchers concluded there was insufficient evidence to suggest outcomes were better with double checking than single.

Koyama, A.K., Maddox, C.S., Li, L., Bucknall, T. & Westbrook, J.I., 2020, 'Effectiveness of double checking to reduce medication administration errors: A systematic review', *BMJ Quality and Safety*, vol. 29, pp. 595–603.

Questions for consideration

- How could findings from this systematic review help to broadly inform evidence-based medication administration practice?
- What future research might be needed to provide sufficient evidence for practice?
- What value can reviews of literature have for other areas of clinical practice?

Activity 9.4   Approaching a literature review

In our case study, April has been asked to undertake a literature review on issues around medication administration by nurses and midwives. She has never written a formal review before and comes to you for advice. Using the knowledge you have gained in this chapter, summarise the information she needs to successfully complete the assessment.

Chapter summary

Literature reviews can provide valuable information with which to inform evidence-based nursing and midwifery practice. This chapter has examined practicalities in performing reviews of the research literature. The importance of refining the research question, carefully developing and managing the search, and planning and writing the review has been examined.

Chapter review questions

- Why is it important for nurses and midwives to be able to write quality literature reviews?
- What are the key aspects to consider in selecting research literature to include in a review?
- What are important factors to consider in writing a literature review?

Questions for discussion

- How can we utilise literature reviews to enhance evidence-based practice?
- What are the key skills needed to produce high-quality literature reviews?
- What might be limitations to the use of literature reviews to inform evidence-based practice?

Questions for personal reflection

- How have you approached writing literature reviews in the past?
- How might you now do that differently?

Useful web resources

Australian Nursing and Midwifery Federation's Nursing and Midwifery Research Policy <http://anmf.org.au/documents/policies/P_Nursing_Midwifery_Research.pdf>.

National Health and Medical Research Council (2016) NHMRC Standards for Guidelines <https://www.nhmrc.gov.au/guidelinesforguidelines/standards>.

US National Library of Medicine's Medical Subject Headings <www.nlm.nih.gov/mesh/>.

References and further reading

Aveyard, H., 2023, *Doing a Literature Review in Health and Social Care: A Practical Guide*, 5th edn, London: Open University Press.

Bell, T., Sprajcer, M., Flenady, T. & Sahay, A., 2023, 'Fatigue in nurses and medication administration errors: A scoping review', *Journal of Clinical Nursing*. doi: 10.1111/jocn.16620.

Cooper, S., Cant, R., Kelly, M., Levett-Jones, T., McKenna, L., Seaton, P. & Bogossian, F., 2021, 'An evidence-based checklist for improving scoping review quality', *Clinical Nursing Research*, vol. 30, no. 3, pp. 230–240.

Koyama, A.K., Maddox, C.S., Li, L., Bucknall, T. & Westbrook, J.I., 2020, 'Effectiveness of double checking to reduce medication administration errors: A systematic review', *BMJ Quality and Safety*, vol. 29, pp. 595–603.

Leite, D.F.B., Padilha, M.A.S. & Cecatti, J.G., 2019, 'Approaching literature review for academic purposes: The literature review checklist', *Clinics*, vol. 74, p. e1403.

Lingard, L., 2017, 'Writing an effective literature review', *Perspectives on Medical Education*, vol. 7, pp. 47–49.

McClatchey, A.K., Shield, A., Cheong, L.H., Ferguson, S.L., Cooper, G.M. & Kyle, G.J., 2018, 'Why does the need for medication become a barrier to breastfeeding? A narrative review', *Women and Birth*, vol. 31, pp. 362–366.

Murad, M.H., 2017, 'Clinical practice guidelines: A primer on development and dissemination', *Mayo Clinic Procedures*, vol. 92, no. 3, pp. 423–433.

Paul, J. & Criado, A.R., 2020, 'The art of writing literature review: What do we know and what do we need to know?', *International Business Review*, vol. 29, article 101717.

Pollock, D., Davies, E.L., Peters, M.D.J., Tricco, A.C., Alexander, L., McInerney, P., Godfrey, C.M., Khalil, H. & Munn, Z., 2020, 'Undertaking a scoping review: A practical guide for nursing and midwifery students, clinicians, researchers, and academics', *Journal of Advanced Nursing*, vol. 77, pp. 2102–2113.

Silva, A.R., Padilha, M.I., Petry, S., Silva, V.S.E., Woo, K., Galica, J., Wilson, R. & Luctkar-Flude, M., 2022, 'Reviews of literature in nursing research: Methodological considerations and defining characteristics', *Advances in Nursing Science*, vol. 45, no. 3, pp. 197–208.

US National Library of Medicine, 2023, *Medical Subject Headings*, <https://www.nlm.nih.gov/mesh/meshhome.html>.

10 Sharing research

Learning objectives

After working through this chapter, you should be able to:

- Discuss the importance of disseminating nursing and midwifery research
- Compare and contrast different methods through which nursing and midwifery research can be shared
- Discuss key principles underpinning professional dissemination of research
- Identify ways by which the impact of research can be optimised

Key terms and concepts

Abstract, citations, conference, dissemination, impact, metrics, presentation skills, writing for publication.

Case study overview

In Chapter 6, we introduced you to Alice, a clinical nurse specialist, who was concerned that deterioration of patients on her ward was not being identified early. She set about developing a scoping review on the topic to see what could be implemented to improve this. On completion of her review, Alice knew that it was important for her to share what she had found.

Chapter introduction

Sharing, or *dissemination*, of research findings is arguably the most important part of the research process. As part of your research, you may have depended on people to participate in activities such as interviews, focus groups or surveys. You will also have provided them with information prior to participation outlining how you will share your findings and this will likely have been also outlined in your ethics application. Combined with this, participants will have given valuable time and information to enable you to complete your work. In this sense, you have an obligation to report your research findings. On completion of your study, you will have important findings but how broadly and effectively they are implemented will depend on the ways by which you communicate them. This chapter explores different ways to disseminate your important research findings professionally and in a way that optimises the impact of your research.

DOI: 10.4324/9781003414476-14

Presenting your work

There is a variety of ways by which you can share your important research findings. This might be locally to colleagues or fellow students, or more formally via seminars or conference presentations. In this section, we will look at some of the practicalities in presenting your work.

Conferences

Conferences provide fora that facilitate sharing of research and scholarship among like-minded peers. They provide opportunities for networking with people who share your research interests, and with colleagues who may subsequently implement your research findings. Presenting at relevant national or international conferences is a great way to present your work; however, both preparation and planning required for success. Nursing and midwifery conferences are usually run by professional organisations with either a general or specific focus. They are generally organised well in advance of the actual conference dates, and a call for abstracts will be circulated by the organising or scientific committee anywhere up to 12 months prior, so you need to watch carefully for these. Unfortunately, today there are scam conferences advertised so it is important to verify that the one you want to attend is real. Look carefully to ensure the organisation hosting the conference is legitimate.

A call for **abstracts** will generally provide guidance about the specific topics or themes being focused on for the conference and the guidelines for preparing an abstract; sometimes there will even be a template that needs to be utilised. There is usually a non-negotiable closing date for abstracts. The abstract presents an overview of your research and what you want to present and will be considered by the conference's scientific committee who will decide whether or not to accept it for presentation.

Abstracts are short summaries of your research and often have a word limit around 250 or 300 words in total. Your abstract needs to tell the entire story about your research. Hence, the key components of an abstract usually include the following:

- One or two sentences on the background to the study and the need for doing the study
- One sentence stating the study aim or objective
- A sentence detailing the study methodology, another describing the methods and participants
- One or two sentences describing the key findings
- One or two sentences providing an interpretation of the findings and recommendations
- A concluding sentence

Generally, there should be no abbreviations or references in an abstract, unless specifically indicated in the guidelines. Some conferences have very strict requirements for the content of abstracts, while others are more relaxed. For some, the results must be finalised at the time of writing the abstract and the final presentation must match the abstract (this is particularly important if prizes will be awarded). Others allow a vague statement of results in the abstract, such as 'results will be presented'. It is important to read the guidelines carefully. Tables 10.1 and 10.2 provide examples of unstructured and structured abstracts.

Table 10.1 Sample unstructured abstract

Contemporary nursing and midwifery education: challenges and opportunities
The professions of nursing and midwifery have evolved significantly in recent decades and
continue to develop. Like knowledge in other fields, the knowledge underpinning clinical
practice changes rapidly. With this come new technologies to assist in the provision of health
care which nurses and midwives need to be able to utilise effectively. Increasing focus on
patient safety and quality, along with better informed consumers, means that they must be
increasingly knowledgeable and accountable and use evidence to support their practice, as well
as generate knowledge to inform clinical practice. Nurses and midwives must also have skills
to participate effectively within interprofessional teams. Issues such as globalisation of the
workforce and generational change further pose new challenges in maintaining a responsive
and well-educated workforce. This presentation will explore these issues in the context of the
need to provide contemporary education in order to meet changing health care environments
and ensure optimal patient and community health outcomes. It will also introduce some of the
educational models emerging in response to such changes.

Table 10.2 Sample structured abstract

Listening style preference of first year undergraduate nursing and midwifery students
Background: Effective communication is fundamental to nursing and midwifery practice
and listening is considered an essential communicative function. Despite the importance of
listening as a core communication function, few studies have explored the listening preference
of first-year undergraduate students.
Aim: The aim of the study was to explore the listening style preference of first-year
undergraduate nursing and midwifery students.
Method: This was a cross-sectional study using a validated tool. At the end of a lecture,
students were invited to participate in the study by a research member not directly involved
in students' teaching. They were provided with an explanatory statement and informed that
participation was voluntary and anonymous.
Results: A total of 205 first-year students completed the survey, representing 67% response
rate. Participants were predominately female and in the age group, less than 25 years. Strong
preference was noted among the students for the People listening style and least preference
for Action-oriented listening style. No significant difference in listening preference styles was
found between sexes.
Conclusion: People listening style is concerned about emotions and feelings of others. The
strong preference for this style is consistent with career choice for this cohort of students.
Educational interventions should focus on all styles, with recognition of preference in this
group.

After a period of time, you will receive notification of whether or not your abstract has
been accepted for presentation. There are a variety of presentation modes possible, but
the most common are podium/oral presentations and poster presentations. Oral presentations are usually done in front of an audience, in person, online or in **hybrid** mode,
the latter becoming very popular as a result of COVID-19 limitations on travel. Poster
presentations allow you to present your research on a poster. While generally these are
physical posters, some conferences offer opportunities for these also to be delivered virtu-
ally. Once accepted, you will receive specific guidelines on preparing your presentation
for the specific conference. However, there are key principles that apply to any type of
presentation that should be considered.

Preparing presentations

Oral or podium conference presentations are usually 15–20 minutes in duration and your presentation will be one of a group of presentations in a session. However, similar considerations need to be given to presentation to other groups such as peers in health care or education settings. Most often, people use Microsoft Powerpoint® to prepare these.

It is important to ensure that whatever type of presentation you are doing, it is professional and reflects both yourself and your organisation in a positive way. You can think about it as a form of advertising for yourself or your organisation.

First, you need to identify a suitable **template**. Most health care and education institutions have their own corporate template which is best to use. However, regardless of the template used, there are key principles that need to be considered. It is important that the presentation supports you, not replaces what you have to say. They should provide visual information while the focus still remains on you as the presenter. So, in developing your materials, consider the following:

- Work on the principle of one slide per minute at the most in your presentation.
- Keep slide content to a minimum, only short, concise bullet points or graphics.
- Avoid clutter on slides and carefully consider the style for presenting the content on each.
- Have one key idea or area of focus on each slide.
- Ensure the font is large enough for the audience to read easily and that font is consistent across all slides.
- Ensure that graphics are clear and sharp.
- Ensure that any ideas or content you use are appropriately cited, including images sourced from websites.

Given the focus is on you and not your presentation slides, you need to think about how you are seen by others. You want to engage your audience and be confident in delivering your content. **Rehearsal** is imperative to ensure you can do this well. Consider recording yourself and watching it back. Note your mannerisms and ways in which you could develop your presenting skills. Box 10.1 offers some practical suggestions for delivering successful and professional presentations.

Box 10.1   Presentation tips

- Use cue cards as prompts with key points to cover, do not read off your slides or written script. You want to engage with your audience and appear natural in your presenting.
- Keep regular eye contact with, and across your audience, throughout the presentation.
- Speak confidently and ensure that the tone of your voice varies. Avoid words such as 'um' or 'and so on'.
- Short pauses in some places can help the audience to digest your content and allow you to think about what to say next.
- Rehearse and check timings several times before the scheduled presentation and ensure your body language is relaxed and engaging. Consider recording your practice and watching it back.
- Breathe deeply and relax!

Activity 10.1   Think about a presentation you have given in the past

How did that align with the tips provided in Box 10.1? What did you do well? How well did you engage the audience? What could you have done differently?

Activity 10.2   Now consider Alice in our case study for this chapter

She has decided to begin disseminating her findings by presenting a short education session for staff in her ward. What tips would you give Alice to ensure she delivered a professional presentation that was engaging and encouraged others to be interested in her work?

Writing up and publishing your work

Publishing research work is important for several reasons. It disseminates important research findings and ideas to a wide audience, builds the researcher's professional credibility and profile and contributes to the profession and its knowledge base. Furthermore, you might have told participants and ethics committees how you planned to disseminate your research findings, so you have an ethical responsibility to do this. Yet, many researchers fail to deliver on this. Publishing in journals is not easy and requires careful attention and work but the personal and professional rewards from publication success can be great. If you are new to this, seek out an experienced researcher who can provide you with advice and feedback along the way.

Many people write their manuscripts before they consider where they will publish them. This can be problematic as each journal has specific requirements, readers and focus that need to be considered as you write. Prior to commencing writing for publication, there are some key questions that need to be asked, such as:

- What is new and innovative about my work?
- Who is the audience I am writing for?
- Which journal/s should I publish in?
- Is this the right journal for my work?
- What are the metrics for my chosen journal?
- Is this the right time for my research to be published in this journal?

We will look at each of these in detail.

Audience

Many novice researchers develop manuscripts for journal submission because they are required to, particularly if enrolled in research programs. However, the impact of a publication will come from other researchers reading that work, building upon it and citing it in their own work. They might even use surveys you have developed or want to replicate your approach locally. During the writing process, it is important to consider the audience for whom you are writing. Who is it that you want to read your work? Which journals do those people read and write for? There are so many available journals and this is increasing all the time, so it can take time to find the right one for your audience.

Selecting a suitable journal

Selecting the right journal can be challenging with increasingly differing quality, scope and access options. It is important to initially consider a range of suitable journals from which you can then determine priorities. This section explores some of the considerations in doing this well.

First, explore the journals that are specific to your research topic. With many predatory journals around, it is best to use credible databases, such as Scopus, Web of Science, CINAHL or Proquest to assist with identifying the best journal/s for your work. Try to come up with a list of potential journals that you can assess further. In evaluating potential journals, there are many aspects to consider:

• Look, first, at whether the journal publishes the type of study and manuscript you are wanting to submit. For example, a journal might publish systematic reviews, but not other types of reviews. If author guidelines are not clear, take a careful look at the papers they have published recently.
• Look at the editorial board. Are there notable researchers represented there? Is there a good spread of editors from different countries and your own region?
• Look at the journal's scope. What is the scope of work they publish and how does your work align?
• What are the journal's turnaround times? If your work is new and innovative, you want to get it disseminated fast and before others researching similar topics do.
• Does the journal publish by subscription, open access or a combination of both? Subscription means that only readers who access through a subscription, usually through a library, can access the journal contents. On the other hand, open access journals are available to everyone but often come with a significant fee for the author. Some journals are hybrid in nature, so publish both subscription for free and open access for a fee. How you choose to publish will likely be influenced by whether or not you have the funds to spend on open access options.
• Consider what the journal has previously published around your topic. Is there a way you can demonstrate that your work builds upon that? Has the journal recently published similar work to yours? If so, they may not be interested in your work, rather looking for new and novel work.
• What are the journal's metrics? In Chapter 6, we introduced the concept of metrics, including impact factor. The higher the impact factor, the more likely your work is going to be cited. Nursing and midwifery journals have lower impacts than some other scientific journals. Is your work applicable beyond nursing or midwifery? If so, there may be relevant journals with higher impact factors outside the profession that are worth considering. You should always seek to get the best impact for your work. However, sometimes that impact might not be measured by metrics. Your work might be suitable to a small specialist audience that can only be reached through a professional, rather than academic, journal.
• Is there an upcoming special issue being published by a journal that matches your work? It can take time to get manuscripts into press but for special issues, the process can be expedited, meaning your work becomes available to others quicker. This can be important if you are seeking to disseminate your work quickly.

> ### Activity 10.3   Select three journals relevant to your area of interest
>
> Explore their author guidelines and metrics. How would you evaluate which one might be the best journal in which to try to publish? Why?

Preparing the manuscript

Once you have identified a journal that suits your work, it is important to ensure that your work fits the journal's aim and scope. Ensuring that your work is suitable will increase the likelihood of the manuscript progressing through initial checking and onto an editor for consideration. In writing the manuscript, be clear about the message you want the manuscript to tell and highlight the innovation or new knowledge being presented. Editors want to publish new ideas or innovative angles to existing ones.

Before submitting your manuscript, carefully review the journal's **author guidelines**. Each will have its own, sometimes very specific requirements that must be followed. Not conforming to these might mean the paper is rejected even before being sent onto an editor for consideration. Check also the language, grammar and spelling that are appropriate for the journal. Many English-language journals use specific spelling such as UK or US English. If the author guidelines are unclear on this, review a recently published paper in the journal and check the style. Finally, check if there is a specific referencing style used in the journal and ensure your paper is prepared accordingly. Many good manuscripts do not even make the review process because they have not been prepared according to a journal's requirements. Carefully also check whether the journal has other specific requirements that need to be addressed.

In developing the manuscript, begin by structuring the paper exactly as the journal requires it. Many journals are specific about things such as how sections are titled, use of capital letters and referencing style. In addition, some have structured abstracts with sub-headings, while others do not. Regardless, prepare the abstract using the guidelines presented earlier in this chapter.

When you submit your paper, you will be asked to use keywords. Many authors underestimate the importance of these. With rapid growth of reviews, such as scoping, systematic and rapid reviews, optimising the likelihood of your work being identified for inclusion could depend on the keywords you choose. The National Library of Medicine in the United States provides a comprehensive site for Medical Subject Headings (MeSH) that is regularly updated and should be used as the first strategy in developing keywords for your manuscript. This can be accessed at: https://www.nlm.nih.gov/mesh/meshhome.html.

Authorship

Authorship is an important consideration. Being an author brings credit, but it also brings responsibility and accountability for what is published. Too often, people are named as authors but have not made sufficient contributions to warrant this level of recognition. An 'author' is generally considered to be someone who has made substantial intellectual contribution to the design of a study, data collection and analysis. For manuscripts that will have more than one author, decisions about who will be authors and the order of authors should be made before starting to write up the work. Increasingly, journals are requiring that authorship conforms to the International Committee of Medical Journal Editors' guidelines for authorship. It is useful to consult these prior to commencing writing; they can be located at: https://www.icmje.org/recommendations/browse/

roles-and-responsibilities/defining-the-role-of-authors-and-contributors.html. Where there are contributors who do not meet the criteria for authorship, the acknowledgement section is a great place to acknowledge those people who have helped with the work.

The review process

Once your manuscript has been submitted to a journal for consideration, the process can be lengthy. However, a manuscript can only be considered by one journal at a time. Under no circumstances should a manuscript be submitted to more than one journal for consideration at the same time.

Initially, your manuscript will be checked by the journal's editorial office to ensure all required documents are submitted and the manuscript has been prepared according to the author guidelines. Once passing through initial checking, it will move to an Editor who will make several considerations, such as the alignment of the work with the journal, whether the work would be relevant and interesting to the journal's readers, whether it builds on previous work the journal has published, and importantly, whether it makes a new contribution to knowledge in the field. At this point, the Editor will either reject the work or send it out for peer review. There are different approaches to peer review, depending on the individual journal, namely:

- **Blind review**—The author/s and reviewers are not identified to each other during the process, and reviewers will not be identified later.
- **Open review**—The authors and reviewers are identified to each other from the beginning.

For most journals, there are at least two reviewers for each manuscript. They will review the work and make a recommendation to the Editor. If there is significant discrepancy between their reviews, the Editor may invite a third reviewer. It is becoming increasingly challenging for Editors to secure sufficient reviewers for manuscripts and common to invite many potential reviewers before securing sufficient numbers. This is making the process lengthier than in the past and requiring authors to be patient.

Once sufficient reviews have been returned, the Editor will make a final decision on the work which will be:

- accept without amendments (This is very uncommon)
- minor revisions
- major revisions
- reject

If the reviewers and Editor see sufficient potential in the paper, they will ask for revisions. If major, this will usually require another round of review, further lengthening the process. However, if you can address their comments suitably, it can result in success.

Manuscripts can be rejected for many reasons. These may be related to the work itself or challenges with the journal. It is important to consider the common reasons why manuscripts are rejected to give your work the best possible chance of being accepted. These include:

- The research design or reporting is of poor quality.
- The manuscript development is inadequate or author guidelines have not been followed.
- The work is presented with poor English language and/or grammar.
- The work does not fit the journal well.
- The journal has recently published similar work, or has similar work under consideration or in press, and the submission does not offer anything new.
- There is nothing new or innovative in the work presented.
- The journal has too many papers to consider.

Activity 10.4   Again, consider Alice in our case study for this chapter

After presenting her work to her peers, one suggested that Alice attempt to publish her review. Not having been through this process before, how would you recommend Alice go about doing this? How could she identify where to publish her work?

Research Example 10.1   Increasing publication rates

Writing research findings up for journal publication is important to ensure others can learn from and use them, and as we identified earlier, is an ethical responsibility. However, much important research is never disseminated. At one large academic medical centre in the United States, a 12-week writing for publication workshop was designed for 89 nurses and each was matched with a mentor (Fischer-Cartlidge, 2020). This, up to the time of publication, had resulted in 29 manuscripts being submitted and at various stages of review. In the program evaluation, 84% of participants reported that they were likely or very likely to write again for publication, and 96% reported improved writing skills (Fischer-Cartlidge, 2020).

Fischer-Cartlidge, E., 2020, 'An evidence-based approach to increasing nurses' publication rates', *AJN*, vol. *120*, no. *8*, pp. 50–55.

Questions for consideration

- What skills could nurses or midwives require to publish their research findings?
- What strategies could be employed in organisations to improve writing skills and publication outputs?

Research Example 10.2   Measuring research outputs

Increasingly, emphasis is being placed on the application of research findings to enable quality evidence-based practice and ultimately, quality patient outcomes. Contributing knowledge to the evidence base is an important consideration for nurses and midwives. In France, Goyet et al. (2018) conducted a survey with midwives around their experiences and perceptions of research and publication. They also undertook a **bibliometric analysis** of their publications. At the time, there were 146 midwives in the country with master's or PhD qualifications and/or had published in scientific or professional journals. The researchers identified 218 publications from these midwives, with 89 being directly related to midwifery practice or interventions. Pregnancy and birth were the topics most commonly covered. Their analysis indicated that publication by midwives was increasing each year.

Goyet, S., Sauvegrain, P., Schantz, C. & Morin, C., 2018, 'State of midwifery research in France', *Midwifery*, vol. 64, pp. 101–109.

Questions for consideration

- What does this research indicate about growing awareness of publication?
- What limitations might there be for nurses and midwives to publish their research work? How might these be overcome?

After successfully publishing your work

Having your work published is very exciting but many researchers treat this as the final part of disseminating their research. However, it is only one step in a longer process. Having your work cited by other researchers is important for a number of reasons. For a researcher, citations contribute to one's h-index, a measure of the impact of one's work that we introduced in Chapter 6. It also indicates that it has been read and built upon (Watson et al., 2019).

With increasingly large numbers of journal publications each year, it is no longer feasible to read every paper published in one's area of interest. Having strategies for increasing the likelihood of people noticing your work is now important. Social media has become a vital part of how authors now achieve this. On publication of your work, most journals will send you links for Facebook, Twitter and LinkedIn to advertise your work throughout your networks. There are also scholarly collaboration networks that are useful for researchers sharing their work including ResearchGate, Academia.edu and Mendeley. Using such platforms to let others know about your research will build your profile and citations, encourage other researchers with similar interests to contact you and promote collaboration and, finally, increase the potential implementation of your findings.

Chapter summary

Undertaking research in nursing and midwifery is vital for building the knowledge base for the professions. Research findings can be shared in a multitude of ways through formal and informal networks to optimise impact. This chapter has highlighted how research can be communicated professionally through presentation and publications, along with the increasingly important role that social media plays in sharing research.

Chapter review questions

- Why is it important to disseminate nursing and midwifery research?
- What methods can be used to share research outcomes?
- What are key considerations in presenting nursing and midwifery research?
- What should researchers consider in preparing research manuscripts?
- How can social media assist with nursing and midwifery research dissemination?

Questions for discussion

- What role does ethics play in the dissemination of nursing and midwifery research?
- What challenges might nurse or midwife researchers encounter in the publication process? How might these be managed?
- What are the implications in publishing research in professional journals as opposed to academic journals?

Questions for personal reflection

- How well developed are your presentation skills? How might you develop these further?
- How would you describe your professional writing skills? What aspects could you work to develop further?

Useful web resources

International Committee of Medical Journal Editors (2023) Defining the Role of Authors and Contributors <https://www.icmje.org/recommendations/browse/roles-and-responsibilities/defining-the-role-of-authors-and-contributors.html>.
National Library of Medicine (2022) Welcome to Medical Subject Headings (MeSH) <https://www.nlm.nih.gov/mesh/meshhome.html>.

References and further reading

Astroth, K.S. & Hain, D., 2019, 'Disseminating scholarly work through nursing presentations', *Nephrology Nursing Journal,* vol. 46, no. 5, pp. 545–549.
Bellquist, J.E., 2021, 'Reporting nursing research, an essay on style: Beginnings', *Nurse Author & Editor,* vol. 31, no. 1. pp. 10–12.
Carter-Templeton, H., 2021, 'Writing productivity strategies', *Nurse Author & Editor,* vol. 31, no. 2, pp. 33–35.
Chicca, J. & Chunta, K. 2020, 'Developing ideas for publication: Strategies for nurse authors', *Nurse Author & Editor,* vol. 30, no. 2, pp. 1–11.
Fischer-Cartlidge, E., 2020, 'An evidence-based approach to increasing nurses' publication rates', *AJN,* vol. 120, no. 8, pp. 50–55.
Goyet, S., Sauvegrain, P., Schantz, C. & Morin, C., 2018, 'State of midwifery research in France', *Midwifery,* vol. 64, pp. 101–109.

McKenna, L., Cooper, S., Cant, R. & Bogossian, F., 2017, 'Editorial: Research publication performance of Australian Professors of Nursing & Midwifery', *Journal of Advanced Nursing*, doi: 10.1111/jan.13338.

McKenna, L. & Gray, R., 2018, 'Editorial: The importance of ethics in research publications', *Collegian*, vol. 25, pp. 147–148.

Ryan, R. & Sfar-Gandoura, H., 2018, 'Disseminating research information through Facebook and Twitter (DRIFT): Presenting an evidence-based framework', *Nurse Researcher*, vol. 26, no. 1, pp. 41–49.

Saver, C., 2022, 'From poster to publication: Seven steps to success', *Nurse Author and Editor*, vol. 32, no. 1, pp. 8–10.

Siedlecki, S.L., 2022, 'Presenting your research findings: Tips from a conference chair', *Clinical Nurse Specialist*, vol. 36, no. 5, pp. 233–240.

Stucky, C.H., 2020, 'Advancing nursing leadership through writing: Strategies for publishing success', *Journal of Continuing Education in Nursing*, vol. 51, no. 10, pp. 447–449.

Watson, R., 2020, 'The contribution of peer review to scholarly publishing', *Nurse Author & Editor*, vol. 30, no. 2, pp. 1–6.

Watson, R., McKenna, H. & Thompson, D., 2019, 'Increasing citations to your work', *Journal of Advanced Nursing*, vol. 755, pp. 1601–1603.

Section 5

How Do I Pursue a Nursing or Midwifery Research Future?

So far in this book, we have focused on understanding research and its application to nursing and midwifery through evidence-based practice. However, increasingly, nurses and midwives are driving research projects and the generation of quality knowledge to support practice. Many do this as part of their clinical or academic roles, while others seek to pursue a purely research-focused role, specialising in the generation of new knowledge. So, while you may be thinking about what type of clinical role you would like to focus on in your future career, research is a pathway. This section, consisting of one final chapter, introduces various options for research careers in nursing and midwifery. It examines different educational pathways to research careers, whether these be clinically or academically focused.

Increasingly, nurses and midwives are seeking ways to attract funding, small and large, to support their research activity. This might be for a small research project in a single ward area or a large, multi-centre clinical trial. The skill of writing research proposals is important to success. Some undergraduate and postgraduate courses include the writing of research proposals, so in the second part of this section, we present a step-by-step approach to developing your own quality research proposal.

DOI: 10.4324/9781003414476-15

11 Research pathways for nurses and midwives

Learning objectives

After working through this chapter, you should be able to:

- Define the term *clinical trial*
- Identify research roles that nurses and midwives can undertake
- Discuss the role played by the research nurse or research midwife
- Identify research pathways for nurses and midwives
- Explore opportunities for seeking funding for research ideas
- Identify the key components of a research proposal
- Write a quality research proposal

Key terms and concepts

Clinical doctorate, clinical trial nurse, evidence generator, funding, midwife researcher, nurse researcher, research degree, research midwife, research nurse, research proposal.

Case study overview

Li is a clinical nurse specialist working in a busy women's health unit. She is really interested in getting involved in research, having completed a master's degree and undertaken a small research project as part of her studies. An opportunity has arisen for Li to take on a role as a clinical research nurse in a newly funded project being undertaken by a group of researchers exploring the effectiveness of a newly available drug for managing the effects of early menopause. She decides that this is a great opportunity to develop her research skills so agrees to take up the role.

Chapter introduction

Research plays an important role in the everyday lives of all nurses and midwives in the delivery of effective and evidence-based care. However, the use and conduct of research in nursing and midwifery can be much broader than merely implementing the findings of others' research into practice. While many nurses choose to specialise within the vast array of clinical specialty areas, there are many ways in which nurses and midwives can also be active in the generation of research and even specialise in research roles. Some of

DOI: 10.4324/9781003414476-16

these are clinically based, while others are more distant from the bedside. In this chapter, we will explore research roles in the two disciplines, including the possible pathways to a research career.

Increasingly, there is an expectation that midwives and nurses in clinical practice roles will engage with research findings, to underpin their practice, as well as in the generation of research studies. Sometimes, there are opportunities to apply for funding to support engagement in research activities, so skills in writing funding proposals are important. In the second half of the chapter, we will explore the fundamental aspects of developing a research proposal, either for the purposes of further studies or for attracting funding to support research activities.

Evidence generator: the nurse/midwife as researcher

Throughout this text, we have introduced basic concepts underpinning research, including approaches to doing research and to critiquing and utilising the research conducted by others. However, increasingly, there are specific research roles for nurses and midwives, particularly in clinical settings. These offer unique opportunities for individuals interested in pursuing research careers, including for the **research nurse** or **research midwife**, nurse or midwife researcher and academic researcher.

Research nurse or midwife

Research roles for nurses and midwives are growing. One role that is not well written about is that of the research nurse or midwife. Also known as *clinical research nurses*, *clinical trial nurses* or *clinical research midwives*, they play an important role in managing funded research projects, specifically **clinical trials**—that is, studies that seek to examine the effectiveness of new treatments in clinical practice with a view to enhancing or changing the management of patients. Research nurses and midwives are employed in research-specific locations or on research projects for the duration of a funded study. However, as demonstrated in Research Examples 11.1 and 11.2, there is a move towards nurses and midwives leading the design and implementation of their own clinical trials.

Globally, numbers of clinical trials are growing, and, thus, the demand for research nurses—and, to a lesser extent, research midwives—has grown. Clinical trials are common for testing new medications, medical devices or changes in usual approaches to care. To ensure they are of the highest quality, clinical trials are conducted in a very rigorous way and often involve a number of professionals, such as doctors, nurses, midwives, pharmacists and allied health professionals.

Research nurses and midwives undertake a variety of roles in clinical trials. Traditionally, these have been very limited, such as collecting samples, in the actual research process. However, the roles have expanded significantly, and many other activities are now commonly undertaken by research nurses and midwives, such as:

- managing projects from beginning to end;
- recruiting participants, usually patients or other healthcare consumers;
- communicating with other health professionals, project team members and relevant authorities related to the study;

- managing data collection, which might include taking samples (for example, blood or urine) or monitoring (for example, blood pressure);
- entering data into computer programs or project paperwork;
- contributing to the development of new treatments (for example, new medications);
- working within a multidisciplinary team that may include doctors, pharmacists, allied health professionals and scientists;
- interacting with patient participants, including coordinating appointments and clinical procedures;
- monitoring the effects of interventions (for example, new treatments);
- identifying and reporting adverse events;
- ensuring the safety of participants;
- ensuring the study adheres to study protocols and ethical and legislative requirements;
- submitting project reports and
- promoting research awareness and research culture among key stakeholders.

In the United Kingdom, Kunhunny and Salmon (2017) undertook a study to explore the professional identity of the clinical research nurse. They interviewed 11 clinical research nurses about their roles and professional identities. The findings indicated that the nurses were very satisfied with their ability to act as 'agents of change in health care' through their research engagement.

While previously most clinical trials were medically led, there is now a growing focus on increasing nurse- and midwife-led clinical trials directed towards further improving patient care and practice. To enable this to flourish, developing strong research culture in the clinical space and empowering nurses to undertake research has been recognised as important (O'Brien et al., 2022). Established in 2020, the Australasian Nursing and Midwifery Clinical Trials Network is working to contribute to this by promoting research collaborations, resource sharing, training and strengthening development of grant applications.

Activity 11.1　Exploring the clinical research nurse role

In this chapter's case study, Li has agreed to take on a clinical research nurse role in a project exploring the effectiveness of a new drug for managing the effects of early menopause. List the types of activities Li may be required to undertake as part of this role.

Nurse or midwife researcher

There are a number of models by which **nurse researchers** and **midwife researchers** may work in research. Often, they work in academic or clinical settings, or both, on studies focused on issues or care aspects that particularly concern nursing or midwifery. Hence, they usually contribute knowledge to the nursing or midwifery disciplines. It is increasingly common for nurse or midwife researchers to design and conduct their own projects, as opposed to working in clinical research teams. These research roles can be combined with academic teaching roles or can be standalone research positions.

Research Example 11.1   Nurse-led clinical trials

The number of clinical trials conducted around the world is growing, however, only recently have nurses begun to lead their own clinical trials. In Ireland, O'Brien et al. (2022) undertook a qualitative study exploring the experiences of a nursing team who implemented an international nurse-led clinical trial testing an advanced symptom management system using mobile device technologies. Focus groups were conducted with 18 nurses from the team then transcribed and thematically analysed. Five themes emerged: *Previous experience of and attitudes to participation in clinical research*, *Decision-making regarding participation in the clinical trial*, *Facilitators of participation in the clinical trial*, *Challenges of research in nursing practice*, and *Future orientation towards research*. Overall, they identified a number of challenges and facilitators but recognised the importance to nursing practice and patient care improvements.

O'Brien, C., Furlong, E., Coughlan, B., Fox, P. & Darley, A., 2022, 'Building research capacity and culture: Exploring nurses' experience of implementing a nurse-led clinical trial', *Journal of Nursing Management*, vol. 30, pp. 1002–1010.

Questions for consideration

• What does the research suggest about the potential importance of nurse-led clinical trials?
• What types of expertise might be important for nurses or midwives leading such trials?

Research Example 11.2   Midwife-led clinical trials

There is a growing focus on midwifery-led clinical research, particularly clinical trials aiming to improve the care of childbearing women and their newborns. In an effort to determine current scope of midwife-led clinical trials, Homer et al. (2023) conducted a scoping review of midwife-led trials reported between 2000 and 2021 in Australia and New Zealand. Using the Australian and New Zealand Clinical Trials Registry, they identified 50 midwife-led trials and 35 peer-reviewed reports. Rating the quality of studies, they concluded most were moderate to high quality. Study quality was an identified issue due to difficulties in blinding participants. They recommended midwives be provided with support to design and conduct trials, as well as to publish their outcomes.

Homer, C., Neylon, K., Kennedy, K., Baird, K., Gilkison, A., Keogh, S., Middleton, S., Gray, R., Whitehead, L., Finn, J., Rickard, C., Sharplin, G., Neville, S. & Eckert, M., 2023, 'Midwife led randomised controlled trials in Australia and New Zealand: A scoping review', *Women and Birth*. doi: 10.1016/j.wombi.2023.03.003.

Questions for consideration

- What does the research suggest about the potential importance of midwife-led clinical trials?
- What types of expertise might be important for midwives leading such trials?

Education pathways to research roles in nursing and midwifery

Growing recognition of the role of nurses and midwives in research-related activity has led to a growth in the need for higher level education and research preparation. While at an undergraduate level, students learn about the role of research, types of studies and how to interpret and implement research into practice, higher degree courses give nurses and midwives the opportunity to develop skills in doing research, so that they can become researchers, in clinical, academic or other settings, and contribute to the knowledge base in their specific discipline. While there is a variety, all higher degree courses, or **research degrees**, require students to undertake some research. People are often fearful of this, as they feel unprepared to carry out their own research. However, it is important to recognise that all of these pathways are designed to provide research training—that is, learning to do research. If you choose to take up such an option, you are not expected to work alone but will have the support and guidance of at least one academic mentor who will work with you throughout the study.

Honours degrees

An honours degree is an undergraduate award offered by many universities to highly achieving students. It is the equivalent of one academic year and commonly provides students with grounding in research methods and the opportunity to complete a small-scale research study under the supervision of academic staff. Honours degrees can provide direct entry into doctoral studies if the grades achieved meet individual university entrance requirements. Sometimes, honours degrees are integrated into graduate nurse or midwife programs.

Research Example 11.3   Honours degrees in Australia

Honours degrees have been offered in Australia for many years as pathways to postgraduate, or higher degree, studies. Traditionally, they involve carrying out a small research study and submission of a thesis or report. Halcomb et al. (2018) conducted a survey of coordinators of nursing honours programs across Australia. Fifteen respondents reported on their honours programs. The researchers identified variety in the types of programs offered and in the assessment requirements. They also found that there was a perception that honours degrees were not often valued in clinical practice. However, they stressed that the value in honours degrees is their potential to steer students towards leadership roles in nursing, as well as towards doctoral studies.

E. Halcomb, E. Smyth, L. Moxham, V. Traynor & R. Fernandez, 2018, 'Bachelor of Nursing Honours programs in Australia: Trends and key challenges', *Collegian*, vol. 25, no. 4, pp. 429–434.

Questions for consideration

- What are some of the issues associated with honours degrees?
- What factors would impact on your consideration of studying for an honours degree?
- How could honours degrees benefit clinical practice?

Master's degrees

Most universities offering nursing or midwifery courses also offer master's degrees. There is a variety of these on offer; some consist of all coursework, others offer coursework as well as a small-scale research study and others can be done purely by conducting and reporting on a research study. Coursework components can be generic or pathways to specialised practice, such as intensive care or emergency nursing. Students doing coursework master's degrees who also have the opportunity to undertake a research study should seriously consider doing so, as it may later provide entry pathways into doctoral studies, and it is wise to keep future employment and study options open.

Doctor of Philosophy

The Doctor of Philosophy (or PhD) is a postgraduate degree which in many countries entirely consists of a large research study; it is the usual pathway for an individual seeking an academic career in a university or as a full-time researcher. At the end of the course, the candidate is required to submit for examination a thesis, usually around 80,000–100,000 words in length. The impetus for research conducted at doctoral level may be a study devised by the student, or the research may form part of a larger study managed by the supervisor.

Professional doctorates

Professional doctorates are gaining popularity in clinical disciplines such as nursing and midwifery, where they are often known as **clinical doctorates** and may also be titled *Doctor of Nursing*, *Doctor of Nursing Practice* or *Doctor of Midwifery*. They were originally introduced to provide entry to advanced practice in health disciplines, such as pharmacy and physiotherapy, and aim largely to develop research skills in clinicians wanting to develop their research knowledge and deliver evidence-based care (Carpenter, 2021). In clinical areas, they are highly valued over the Doctor of Philosophy, which is seen to be more removed from the clinical setting and more academically focused. Professional doctorates usually focus on research that can be translated directly into practice, making a change at the point of care (Rees et al., 2019). They usually consist of some coursework followed by the conduct of a supervised clinical research study and submission of a thesis, usually around 60,000 words in length and are often completed by part-time study to accommodate other employment (Carpenter, 2021).

Activity 11.2   Exploring a research career

In our case study, Li was employed as a research nurse. The funded research project is coming to an end, and she is considering her future professional role. She has enjoyed the research role and decides that she wants to pursue a research career.

Questions for consideration

- What options does Li have for moving in that direction?
- What educational programs could she undertake to support her moving into a research career?

Activity 11.3   Personal reflection

Think about your future direction in nursing or midwifery.

Questions for consideration

- Where do you see yourself working in the next five years?
- How might a research degree help you along that pathway?
- What type of research degree should you be considering given that direction? Why?

Seeking funding for clinical research

One challenge faced by researchers is that of funding their research activity. Funding is used to support the costs of the study, including research assistant salaries, materials for collecting specimens, professional transcription of interview transcripts and equipment, such as computer software and audio-recorders. Fortunately, much of the research undertaken by nurses and midwives does not require extensive funding. Yet, having funding can be the deciding factor in whether a study proceeds or not. Funding can be difficult to source, and funding applications are usually part of a competitive process. There are several options for researchers seeking funding:

- National research organisations (for example, the UK National Institute for Health and Care Research, the Australian Research Council, the Australian National Health and Medical Research Council and the Health Research Council of New Zealand) provide large-scale competitive funding for research conducted by experienced researchers.
- There are many professional nursing and midwifery organisations that provide funding that is often sufficient for small projects conducted by nurses and midwives.
- Specific medical support organisations often have funding rounds to support research related to the condition on which they focus.
- Often, healthcare organisations offer internal funding—small research grants—to support clinicians to undertake research in their clinical areas.
- There are competitive opportunities for researchers to develop their research skills through fellowships that provide supporting salaries for researchers.

Writing a research proposal

Often, writing a research proposal is an assessment requirement for undergraduate or postgraduate research students. While this may feel an onerous task, the ability to write a research proposal is important for any nurse or midwife wanting to influence health care (Clark & Carter, 2019). For example, you may want to conduct a small study in your clinical workplace for which approval needs to be sought or for which you require funding, or you may want to undertake a study as part of a research degree. Strong research proposals are important in the wider competitive area of funding applications. For all of these situations, a research proposal precedes embarking on the study.

A **research proposal** is a blueprint for a planned study. It outlines the background, design, methods and significance of the research. In a competitive environment, a high-quality research proposal can optimise the likelihood of success and ensure a well-managed project that reaches completion. It is important, then, for the proposal to be developed carefully and structured in a logical way. In this section, we will work through the key aspects of writing a high-quality research proposal.

Title

The proposal should begin with a title. This should be clear and concise, so a reader will know exactly what the proposed study is about. Sometimes, the title also contains the type of study being proposed.

Abstract

The abstract presents a brief summary of the proposed research. While it usually appears early in the proposal, it is common for this part to be written after the rest of the proposal has been developed. In general, the abstract should not be more than 300 words in length. It should cover the following information:

- Brief background to the proposed study
- Aim of the research
- Methodology and design for the study
- Location of the study
- Participants in the study
- Data collection, management and analysis approaches
- Potential uses for the findings

Introduction and background

This section should clearly convey to the reader the key focus of your research study and why it is an important study to do. This section should provide a basic introduction to the reader of what your topic is about and the reasons for doing the study. While it may be perfectly clear to you, the reader of your proposal may not be at all familiar with the topic, so this is particularly important if you do not want to lose their interest early on.

Study significance

It is here that you need to demonstrate why your study is necessary and what benefits it will produce. It needs to convince the reader that the study is required and say how the findings will make an impact. It may also be called the *rationale* or *justification* for the study—that is, the reason for the study to be conducted.

Literature review

The literature review provides an overview of the current state of knowledge in your topic. It should provide a summary and a critique of existing research. The idea is to demonstrate a gap in what is currently known, to further justify the need for the study and for your findings, which will fill that gap. The literature review should discuss research no more than five years old to demonstrate the gap in present knowledge. If critical information exists that is older than five years, it should be presented in the background section.

Research problem, aim and question

This section needs to identify the problem to be addressed by the proposed research. The aim of the research is presented as a broad, overarching statement about what the study will set out to do. It is followed by the research question and, in the case of quantitative research, a hypothesis (see Chapter 4).

The research question must be clearly articulated, as it will guide the whole research, and it needs to be written as a question that your research sets out to answer. It is crucial for the research question to be constructed in such a way that it is answerable and realistically able to be researched. In some studies, there will be one main overarching research question which is subdivided into a number of further questions.

Theoretical framework

The theoretical, or conceptual, framework underpinning your research is important. It demonstrates how you are planning to approach the research from a theoretical or philosophical (methodological) position. This is important, as it will guide your research design, data collection and analysis. For example, if you are proposing to do qualitative research, your theoretical framework might be informed by phenomenology or grounded theory. This section may also be conceptually driven, being underpinned by a philosophical position. Whatever your position, it needs to be clearly outlined. This is particularly important when the proposal is being written for academic purposes.

Research design

The research design presents the practicalities of the actual research and constitutes the largest component of the proposal. It should provide a step-by-step description of how the research will actually be carried out. The steps need to align directly with the research aim, research question and theoretical framework. There are numerous categories of information needed here, which are discussed below.

Methods

The methods are the approaches that will be taken to allow the research question to be answered. For example, you might use survey design, semi-structured interviews or observation. There may also be different phases to your study if you are using mixed methods approaches.

Participants

It is essential to identify who the participants will be in your proposed study. Here, there are several questions that need to be answered:

- What will be the participants' particular characteristics?
- How will participants be invited to participate?
- How will they be recruited, and by whom?
- How many participants will be needed?
- Will there be inclusion and exclusion criteria?
- Are they likely to be a vulnerable group? If so, who will need to be involved to ensure they are protected during the research?

Data collection

It is necessary to clarify the nature of the data collection to be employed. Again, it is useful to consider the following:

- Where will the data be collected?
- Who will collect the data?
- How long will the data collection take?

Instruments

The tools you plan to use need to be clearly explained; for example:

- What data collection instruments will be used?
- If they are questionnaires, have they been previously used and shown they are valid and reliable
- If they are qualitative interviews, what questions are to be asked of participants?

In the case of questionnaires, if they have not been validated previously, a pilot study may be needed before the actual study commences, in order for this to be done.

Data management and analysis

How you plan to handle the data when you have them needs to be clearly described. If you will be using quantitative data, this might include information about organising and cleaning up data and entering data into computer programs, along with descriptions of the tests you plan to run. If you will be using qualitative data, you will likely be employing a form of content or thematic analysis, for which there are many approaches, so you will need to describe the steps involved. This includes steps you will take to ensure your interpretations are accurate. Some aspects to consider here include the following:

- What processes will be used for data management?
- Will data be entered into a particular software program?
- How will the data be analysed?
- What tests will be conducted?
- If qualitative data will be collected, how will these be analysed?
- How will rigour in data analysis be achieved? (This is particularly important in qualitative research.)

Ethical considerations

This is a very important section. You need to identify who is required to approve the study, such as hospital managers. If the study will involve people, it will also require the approval of at least one Human Research Ethics Committee. If you are studying at a university and doing clinical research, it is likely that you will need approval from both the university and the hospital. If you are doing a multi-centre study, you may require even more approvals.

This section also needs to clearly outline all the potential ethical issues involved in the conduct of the research. (We covered this in detail in Chapter 7.) It is particularly important to ensure that in your proposal you include the steps you will take to protect the rights of people who are participating in your research.

Timeline

There needs to be a clearly outlined timeline that demonstrates the different activities of the study and when they will occur. It should clearly show the length of the project and when each activity will begin and end. This is an important component for demonstrating that the proposed study is feasible within the suggested timeframe. Often, this information is presented in a visual format in a chart or table.

Budget and resources

Regardless of whether you are formally seeking funding or not, carefully consider how much your proposed study will cost and what resources will be needed to successfully complete it. It is also important in this section to justify why each item is necessary for your project. The budget should be realistic, with accurate and defendable calculations, including other costs such as charges from the university for office space or other organisation-imposed overheads. The types of items to consider here are listed below, followed by examples:

- **Personnel costs** – staff to be employed on the project, such as research assistants
- **Equipment** – digital recorder for qualitative interviews
- **Services** – transcription of qualitative interviews
- **Printing** – questionnaires, consent forms, final reports
- **Travel** – transport to visit participants, usually as costs per kilometre

- **Catering** afternoon tea for focus group participants
- **Room hire** daily room hire for conducting focus groups
- **Dissemination costs** travel to, registration and accommodation for conference attendance to present findings
- **In-kind contributions** equivalent costs for items, such as personnel, that are to be provided free of charge.

Research team

If you propose to lead a team-based project, you will need to provide information on each team member, such as:

- their qualifications and professional affiliations,
- the expertise and previous experience each brings to the research and
- their individual roles in the project.

Dissemination plan

It is useless to do any research without disseminating its findings, so that others can apply them to their own contexts. A research proposal should always include a plan for how the findings will be communicated to others. This might include the following:

- Peer-reviewed international journals, with suggestions of the most relevant journals
- National or international conference presentations, with suggestions of relevant conferences
- Distribution to funding or other professional bodies
- Circulation through social media

We covered this topic in greater detail in Chapter 10.

References

This should contain all of the primary sources used in the proposal.

Appendices

Any supplementary documentation should be presented as appendices.

This might include such things as questionnaires, ethical approvals obtained, letters of support and curricula vitae of the researchers.

Research Example 11.4   A nursing research proposal

In our case study, Li has completed her clinical research nurse role and has decided she would like to conduct her own research studies through enrolling in a Doctor of Philosophy. Her previous research work has sparked an interest in menopause, particularly the experiences of young women having to cope with early menopause. As part of her degree application, she needs to write a proposal. This is what she produces:

Title Young immigrant women's lived experience of early menopause: A phenomenological study

Background Early onset, or premature, menopause is defined as being the onset of menopause prior to the age of 40 years. Besides leading to fertility issues, early menopause can cause a range of medical and psychological issues that necessitate health professional attention. Women experiencing this condition require individualised hormone therapy and counselling (Faubion et al., 2015). Little is known about the experiences of immigrant women experiencing early onset menopause, particularly whether they seek assistance for such issues and whether the existing support mechanisms meet their needs. In addition, it is unclear if there are additional cultural factors that impact on their experience of the condition.

Study significance Early onset menopause is a challenging condition. However, little is known specifically about the experiences of immigrant women with the condition. This study will provide understandings of the issues faced by immigrant women experiencing early menopause so that specifically tailored support and care can be developed.

Literature review The absence of oestrogen caused by early onset menopause can lead to a range of long-term health effects, including cardiovascular disease, neurological disease, osteoporosis, mood, sexual and psychological disorders and premature death (Shuster et al., 2010). A study by Strezova et al. (2017) found that cultural factors influenced the perceptions and experiences of menopause in Macedonian women living in Australia. However, little recent literature could be sourced relating to other immigrant groups. No studies could be sourced that have specifically examined the experiences of immigrant women who have undergone early onset menopause.

Research aim To explore the lived experiences of immigrant women impacted by early onset menopause.

Research question What are the lived experiences of immigrant women with early onset (premature) menopause?

Theoretical framework Phenomenology will underpin the study. This approach aims to reflect the lived experiences of participants and has a long tradition through many philosophers. This research will employ van Manen's (1990) hermeneutic phenomenology. It is a practical approach and allows for insights to be drawn out, along with the meanings and understandings that participants give to their experiences.

Research design Semi-structured interviews will be conducted with approximately fifteen to twenty immigrant women, aged in their twenties or thirties, who have experienced early onset menopause. Women will be recruited by social media (for example, Facebook) and snowball sampling. An interview guide will be developed to guide the interviews. Interviews will be conducted by the student researcher in a quiet and mutually agreed place. Data will be analysed using thematic analysis informed by the work of Braun and Clarke (2006). Themes will be reviewed for accuracy by the research supervisors.

Ethical considerations Women will be provided with verbal information about the study and provide written informed consent prior to undertaking the interview. Confidentiality will be maintained through the use of pseudonyms in reporting the findings. Prior to the interviews, ethical approval to conduct the study will be sought from the university Human Research Ethics Committee.

Timeline

Year 1

January–June Undertake a detailed literature review to inform the study
July–September Refine study, develop interview schedule
October–December Seek ethical approval

Year 2

January–July Recruit participants and conduct interviews
August–December Conduct data analysis

Year 3

January–June Write chapters
July–December Finalise thesis for submission
Budget No funding will be sought for this study. The student researcher will tran-
   scribe the interviews.

References

Braun, V. & Clarke, V., 2006, 'Using thematic analysis in psychology', *Qualitative Research in Psychology*, vol. 3, no. 2, pp. 77–101.
Faubion, S.S., Kuhle, C.L., Shuster, L.T. & Rocca, W.A., 2015, 'Long-term health consequences of premature or early menopause and considerations for management', *Climacteric*, vol. 18, no. 4, pp. 483–491.
Shuster, L.T., Rhodes, D.J., Gostout, B.S., Grossardt, B.R. & Rocca, W.A., 2010, 'Premature menopause or early menopause: Long-term health consequences', *Maturitas*, vol. 65, no. 2, pp. 161–166.
Strezova, A., O' Neill, S., O' Callaghan, C., Perry, A., Liu, J. & Eden, J., 2017, 'Cultural issues in menopause: An exploratory qualitative study of Macedonian women in Australia', *Menopause*, vol. 24, no. 3, pp. 308–315.
van Manen, M., 1990, *Researching Lived Experience: Human Science for an Action Sensitive Pedagogy*, Albany, NY: State University of New York Press.

Questions for consideration

- Is Li's research aim clear?
- Is the research methodology appropriate to the study aim?
- Is the scope of the proposed research activity clear and well outlined?
- Are the proposed data collection and analysis processes appropriate to the chosen methodology?
- Is the timeline for the study realistic?
- Are there aspects that could be further elaborated?

Activity 11.4   Developing a research proposal

Using the research proposal framework provided in the previous section, begin to develop a proposal for a research study that you could undertake.

- What aspects of developing the proposal are particularly challenging?
- Where might you be able to go for support in further developing your proposal?

Additional hints for writing a research proposal

While we have covered the key elements of the research proposal, there are also some helpful hints we suggest you consider before submitting your proposal:

- Remember you are trying to impress the reader, especially if you are seeking funding! Ensure that your proposal looks professional in its appearance and that spelling, grammar and layout are all perfect.
- Ask someone who is unfamiliar with your topic to review the proposal. It needs to sound logical and understandable to someone who does not know the topic as well as you.
- Avoid the use of acronyms. While you know what they mean, the reader may not, and an acronym may mean different things to different people, depending on their context; for example, *PE* may mean *pulmonary embolism* to a nurse but *pre-eclampsia* to a midwife.
- If you are seeking funding, closely review the proposal requirements of the funding agency. Each agency has specific and different requirements.

Chapter summary

Nurses and midwives have increasing opportunities to take on research-focused roles, engaging in the generation of new knowledge to support nursing, midwifery and health care more generally. A variety of research-based courses is available to arm students with the skills needed to engage in research-focused roles, and we have explored many of these in this chapter. The ability to write a quality research proposal is important for nurses and midwives, whether they are engaged in clinical or academic work. We have explored the key components of such a proposal and what each should contain.

Chapter review questions

- What is a clinical trial?
- What research roles are available for nurses and midwives? How do they differ?
- What pathways can nurses and midwives take to pursue research activities?
- Where can nurses and midwives seek funding to support their research?
- What are the key aspects to developing a quality research proposal?

Questions for discussion

- How can nurses and midwives contribute to the generation of research?
- Why should nurses and midwives engage in research activities?
- What are the pathways for nurses and midwives to pursue their research interests?
- What benefits and challenges might be faced by nurses and midwives engaging in research activities?

Questions for personal reflection

- How has your learning in this chapter influenced your perception of research roles in nursing or midwifery?
- Would you consider a future research career? If so, how might you get there?

Useful web resources

Australasian Nursing and Midwifery Clinical Trials Network <https://anmctn.com.au/>.
Australian College of Nursing Foundation Scholarships, Grants and Awards <https://foundation.acn.edu.au/Foundation/grants-awards.aspx>.
Australian Research Council <www.arc.gov.au>.
Health Research Council of New Zealand <https://www.hrc.govt.nz/grants-funding/funding-opportunities>.
International Network for Doctoral Education in Nursing <https://nursing.jhu.edu/excellence/inden/index.html>.
National Health and Medical Research Council <www.nhmrc.gov.au>.
National Institute for Health and Care Research <https://www.nihr.ac.uk/researchers/funding-opportunities/>.
National Institute of Nursing Research <https://www.ninr.nih.gov/>.
Rosemary Bryant Foundation <https://www.rbf.org.au/research/research-grants>.
Royal College of Midwives Research Hub <https://www.rcm.org.uk/promoting/education-hub/research-and-funding/>.
Sigma Nursing Research and Program Grants <https://www.sigmanursing.org/advance-elevate/research/research-grants>.

References and further reading

Ahn, H. & Reifsnider, E., 2021, 'A guide to writing grant proposals for nursing research', *Research in Nursing & Health*, vol. 44, no. 4, pp. 596–597.
Bonnel, W. & Smith, K., 2018, *Proposal Writing for Clinical Nursing and DNP Projects*, 2nd edn, New York: Springer.
Carpenter, J., 2021, 'Professional doctorate in midwifery: What it is and why would I do one?', *The Practising Midwife*, vol. 24, no. 10, pp. 20–24.
Clark, R. & Carter, K.F., 2019, 'Successful grant applications: Follow the 4 F's', *Nursing*, vol. 49, no. 2, pp. 55–58.
Clarke, S.P., 2016, 'Navigating a research-focused doctoral program in nursing', *Nursing Management*, vol. 47, no. 1, pp. 19–20.
Dobrowolska, B., Chruściel, P., Pilewska-Kozak, A., Mianowana, V., Monist, M. & Palese, A., 2021, 'Doctoral programmes in the nursing disipcline: A scoping review', *BMC Nursing*, vol. 20, article 228.

Halcomb, E., Smyth, E., Moxham, L., Traynor, V. & Fernandez, R., 2018, 'Bachelor of nursing programs in Australia: Trends and key challenges', *Collegian*, *vol. 25*, no. 4, pp. 429–434.

Homer, C., Neylon, K., Kennedy, K., Baird, K., Gilkison, A., Keogh, S., Middleton, S., Gray, R., Whitehead, L., Finn, J., Rickard, C., Sharplin, G., Neville, S. & Eckert, M., 2023, Midwife led randomised controlled trials in Australia and New Zealand: A scoping review', *Women and Birth*. doi: 10.1016/j.wombi.2023.03.003.

Jones, H.C., 2015, 'Clinical research nurse or nurse researcher?', *Nursing Times*, vol. *111*, no. 19, pp. 12–14.

Kivunja, C., 2016, 'How to write an effective research proposal for higher degree research in higher education: Lessons from practice', *International Journal of Higher Education*, vol. 5, no. 2, pp. 163–172.

Kunhunny, S. & Salmon, D., 2017, 'The evolving professional identity of the clinical research nurse: A qualitative exploration', *Journal of Clinical Nursing*, vol. 26, pp. 5121–5132.

Lönn, B.B., Hörnsten, Å., Styrke, J. & Hajdarevic, S., 2022, 'Transitioning to the clinical research nurse role: A qualitative descriptive study', *Journal of Advanced Nursing*, vol. 78, pp. 3817–3829.

O'Brien, C., Furlong, E., Coughlan, B., Fox, P. & Darley, A., 2022, 'Building research capacity and culture: Exploring nurses' experience of implementing a nurse-led clinical trial', *Journal of Nursing Management*, vol. *30*, pp. 1002–1010.

Park, H-J. & Yu, S., 2022, 'The role of clinical trial nurses: Transitioning from clinicians to clinical research coordinators', *International Journal of Nursing Practice*, vol. 28, p. e12943.

Perry, A., 2021, 'A research midwife in a pandemic', *British Journal of Midwifery*, vol. 29, no. 2, p. 115.

Rees, S., Ousey, K., Koo, K., Ahmad, N. & Bowling, F.L., 2019, 'Higher degrees in nursing: Traditional research PhD or professional doctorate?', *British Journal of Nursing*, vol. 28, no. *14*, pp. 940–945.

Terrell, S.R., 2023, *Writing a Proposal for Your Dissertation: Guidelines and Examples*, New York: Guildford Press.

Glossary of terms

abstract   a summary of a published article or a conference presentation

action research   a cyclical research approach designed to facilitate change through empowering participants

AGREE   a study reporting guideline for clinical practice guidelines

analysis of variance   a statistical test used for comparing a continuous (ratio or interval) variable between three or more groups; also known as ANOVA

anonymity   the state of a research participant's identity being unknown to researchers

autonomy   the right to exercise one's will

beneficence   to do good; in research, a study should aim to have good potential outcomes

bias   a systematic error in the way participants are selected, outcomes are measured or data are analysed that leads to results being inaccurate

bibliometric analysis   use of statistical measures to analysis publications

blinding or masking   concealment of group allocation from study participants, researchers and others involved in the research or all three

Boolean operator   a term used to combine keywords or search results in specific ways; terms available are *AND*, *OR* and *NOT*

CARE   a study reporting guideline for case reports

case-control design   a non-experimental study design where a group of participants with a certain condition (cases) is studied alongside a similar group of people without the condition (control)

case study   a research approach that examines the complexities of unique stories to explore a particular phenomenon

categorical or nominal data   values that represent a classification or group membership—for example, gender and hair colour

central tendency   a measure, generally towards the middle of a dataset, around which data points are clustered; potential measures are mean, median and mode

CHEERS   a reporting standard for economic evaluations

chi square   a statistical test used for comparing two categorical variables, each of which has two or more values

clinical audit   a review of current practice and performance against best available evidence

clinical doctorate   a clinically focused doctoral degree

clinical practice guidelines   guidelines for informing clinical practice developed from best available evidence

clinical trial   a study that examines the effectiveness of new treatments in clinical practice with a view to enhancing or changing the management of patients

cluster random sampling   a study sampling where selection of participants is by groups rather than individuals

cluster randomised controlled trial   a randomised controlled trial where the unit of randomisation is not the individual participant but a group of participants

coding   a process of marking keywords or phrases in text

coercion   the unethical process of pressurising someone to participate in research

cohort design   a non-experimental study design where participants (the cohort) are studied over a period of time

confidence intervals   parameters between which the true difference between measurements, or effect of an intervention, would lie if it were measured in the whole population

confidentiality   the protection of information that a research participant does not wish to be made public; this can include, but is not limited to, concealment of their identity

confirmability   the degree to which qualitative findings represent participants' perspectives

confounder   a factor not related to an intervention that can influence the outcome being studied

CONSORT   a reporting standard for randomised controlled trials

contamination   a situation where members of a study control group are exposed to the intervention

content analysis   a deductive process of analysing qualitative data; it can be done numerically or in categories

continuity of care   midwifery concept whereby one known midwife, or a small group of midwives, provides care to a woman throughout antenatal, labour, birth and postnatal period

convenience sampling   a sampling method where people are approached because they are readily accessible, and they self-select to take part

correlation   a statistical test used for comparing two continuous variables when both are measured, not manipulated

correlational design   a non-experimental study design in which the aim is to investigate associations between the outcome of interest and other factors

credibility   ensuring interpretations and conclusions drawn from data are truly reflective

Critical Appraisal Skills Programme   a tool for evaluating research quality; also known as CASP

critique   assessment of a research study to identify strengths, weaknesses and quality

cross-sectional design   a non-experimental study design where data are collected at one specific point in time

data   information collected to answer a research question

data analysis   the process of analysing collected data to draw conclusions

data collection   the process of collecting data to answer a research question

database   searchable source of research and grey literature

data extraction   the process of selecting data from studies for inclusion in a systematic or scoping review

data immersion   the process by which the qualitative researcher absorbs themselves in data to extract content and meanings

data saturation   the point in qualitative data collection where no new data are being obtained

Declaration of Helsinki   a set of ethical research principles for human research developed by the World Medical Association

deductive approach   a research approach involving developing and testing a hypothesis

deferred or retrospective consent   formal consent for data to be used after those data have been collected

dependability   the consistency of qualitative findings in other, similar conditions

dependent variable   the outcome of interest in a quantitative study

descriptive qualitative research   a qualitative research approach that seeks to describe a particular phenomenon

descriptive quantitative design   a non-experimental quantitative study design in which the aim is to describe and quantify a concept of interest; sometimes called an exploratory design

descriptive statistics   measures used to summarise raw data

direct quotation   text taken word-for-word from another person's work; this requires the inclusion of quotation marks citation and possibly also the page number of the work from which the words were taken

discourse analysis   a research approach that examines social and political factors that shape the development of certain practices or circumstances

dispersion   a measure of the degree of variability in a dataset; potential measures are variance, standard deviation, range, interquartile range and frequency

dissemination   communication of research findings, for example, through publication or presentation

EQUATOR Network   Enhancing the Quality and Transparency of Health Research Network

ethical approval   a part of the research process that involves seeking formal approval from a Human Research Ethics Committee to conduct a study

ethics   a discipline area concerned with moral values and conduct

ethnography   a research approach that examines cultural patterns existing in a particular group

ethnomethodology   a research approach that examines the ways in which people feel, understand and explain their world

evidence   knowledge derived from systematic research

evidence-based practice   practice informed by best available research evidence, clinical expertise and client preference

exclusion criteria   characteristics that exclude a participant from a study or a study from a review

external validity   the ability to generalise the results of a study beyond the study sample

fittingness or transferability   the capacity for conclusions from qualitative research to have similar meanings to other, similar populations

focus group   a group of people with which an interview is conducted at the same time

frequency   the count of the occurrences of values in a dataset expressed as a number, a percentage or a proportion

GRADE   measure for evaluating quality of evidence, comprising Grading of Recommendations Assessment, Development and Evaluation

grey literature   literature not published in academic sources

grounded theory   a research methodology that examines social processes in order to develop theory

H-index   a measure of a researcher's publication citations

handsearching   manual searching for literature for inclusion in a literature review

hierarchy of evidence   levels of authority attributed to different forms of research evidence

historical research   a research approach that examines the historical development of a particular concept or situation

honours degree   an undergraduate research degree, usually comprising one year of full-time-equivalent study

HREC   *see* Human Research Ethics Committee

Human Research Ethics Committee   a committee that oversees compliance of human research with ethical standards; also known as an HREC

hypothesis   a statement about assumed variable relationships that can be tested

impact factor   a measure of the impact of a journal, relating to citations of the papers that it publishes

implementation science   an emerging scientific field examining implementation of existing evidence into practice and policy

implied consent   agreement to take part can be assumed by an activity, such as filling out a questionnaire

inclusion criteria   characteristics that a potential participant or a study must possess to be included in research or a literature review

independent variable   a specific factor that could influence the study outcome

inductive approach   an interpretive approach that seeks to develop a new theory or model from data, moving from specific observations to make generalisations

inferential statistics   tests carried out on data to determine whether the results can be generalised from the sample to the population

information power   method for ensuring appropriate sample size in qualitative research

informed consent   a person's agreement to be included in research based on full disclosure of what is involved

internal validity   the ability to attribute the outcome of a research study to the effect of the independent variable and not some other factor

interpretive research   qualitative research that seeks to make meaning of a phenomenon

interquartile range   the difference between the 1st and 3rd quartiles; also known as IQR

interval data   values between which distances (intervals) correspond to real, meaningful, consistent differences in the phenomenon being measured—for example, temperature

intervention   a procedure to which research participants are exposed by the researchers rather than by their own choice; the procedure is managed and controlled by the researchers

interview   a method of data collection where data are collected verbally

interview schedule   key questions used for guiding a research interview

justice   the fair treatment of research participants

knowledge translation   the process of translating research knowledge into practice contexts

Likert scale   a rating scale that allows participants to indicate their level of agreement with presented statements

literature review   a synthesis of previously published research conducted on a particular topic

masking   *see* blinding or masking

mean the average of a set of numbers, obtained by summing all the values and dividing by the number of values in the dataset

median the middle value when the values in a dataset are placed in numerical order; if there is an even number of values, the median is calculated by taking the average of the two middle numbers

Medical Subject Headings a thesaurus of terms maintained by the US National Library of Medicine; also known as MeSH

member checking the process of returning to participants to check interpretations made

MeSH *see* Medical Subject Headings

methodology the philosophical beliefs or assumptions that influence a study's design

midwife researcher a midwife who conducts research

mixed methods a research approach involving mixing of more than one research method in one study, usually combining quantitative and qualitative approaches

mode the most frequently occurring value in a dataset

narrative research a research approach that explores the experiences of people through the stories they tell

narrative review *see* traditional narrative review

nominal data *see* categorical or nominal data

non-maleficence to do no harm; in research, a study should not cause harm to participants

non-probability sampling sampling that does not involve random selection

normal distribution symmetrical distribution of data with the majority of data points clustered around the centre; when represented graphically, it forms a bell-shaped curve

Nuremberg Code a set of ethical research principles developed in response to human experimentation during the Second World War

nurse researcher a nurse who conducts research

observation a data collection method where participants are observed in a specific context

opt out consent a mechanism whereby people refuse consent to take part in research, or for information about them to be used in research, before they become eligible for inclusion; if they do not take up this option, they will be included automatically

ordinal data values that are ordered (ranked), but between which the differences cannot be quantified

paradigm a particular viewpoint of the world

paraphrasing rewriting ideas in one's own words

participant observation a data collection method where participants are observed in a specific context

participatory action research a cyclical research approach designed to facilitate change through working with participants as research team members

participatory research qualitative research that actively involves participants in making change

peer review the process of evaluating an article for its suitability for publication. It is usually undertaken by a minimum of two people with expertise in the topic, the methods used or both

percentile the value at or below which lies a certain percentage of values in a distribution

person-centred care care that is focused on the person and in which the person is given autonomy to make decisions about their care

phenomenology a qualitative research methodology that examines human lived experience

photovoice   a qualitative research approach using photographs to present viewpoints from participants' unique worlds

PICO   an acronym used to name the key aspects of a systematic review, usually referring to *population, intervention, comparator* and *outcome*

population   the entire group of people to whom researchers want to apply their findings

power   the likelihood of a test correctly indicating a real effect of an intervention due to sufficient sample size

pre-post test   a study design where measurements are performed before and after an intervention

predatory journal   a non-credible journal that exploits researchers by charging publication fees without providing academic oversight and rigour, such as peer review

primary source   a paper that provides first-hand reporting of a study by the researcher

probability   the likelihood of a result occurring by chance

probability sampling   sampling based on random selection

protocol   *see* review protocol

purposive sampling   a sampling approach involving purposefully selecting research participants

qualitative descriptive research   a qualitative research approach that seeks to describe a particular phenomenon

qualitative research   a research approach, primarily inductive, that seeks to make meaning of human experience

quantitative research   a research approach, largely deductive, that emphasises objective measurement of information and its numerical analysis

quartile ranking   ranking of journals into four categories, where the 1st quartile, or top 25% (Q1), contains the highest-ranking journals

quasi-experimental design   an experimental study design where there is no control group, or allocation is not performed randomly

quota sampling   study sampling where participants are selected until the quota is filled

randomised controlled trial or true experiment   research design that is the most reliable in establishing cause-and-effect relationships, requiring the presence of an intervention, a control group, and random allocation to the experimental and the control groups; also known as RCT

range   the difference between the highest and lowest value in a dataset

rapid review   systematic type review with limited search and inclusion criteria designed for fast implementation

ratio data   values between which the distances are meaningful and consistent; these variables have a *natural zero*, indicating possible absence of the entity (for example, length, duration, weight), and can be multiplied and divided

RCT   *see* randomised controlled trial or true experiment

realist evaluation   an approach to evaluating programs and how they work

regression   a statistical test examining the effect of manipulating one continuous variable (the independent variable) on a continuous outcome variable (the dependent variable)

reliability   the consistency with which a research instrument measures the construct

research aim   what a researcher is seeking to achieve by doing a study

research degree   a degree that entails conducting a research study

research integrity   honesty in research conduct and reporting

research merit   an ethical principle requiring that a research study must have potential benefit and that this benefit can be realised

research midwife   a midwife who works with a team on a clinical trial

research nurse   a nurse who works with a team on a clinical trial

research process   the whole process of conducting research, from the original idea to the dissemination of findings

research proposal   a structured blueprint for a proposed study

research question   the question that a research study is designed to answer

retrospective consent   *see* deferred or retrospective consent

review protocol   a detailed plan for undertaking a systematic or scoping review

sample   the subset of a population selected to take part in the research

sampling   the process of selecting research participants

saturation   *see* data saturation

scoping review   a structured literature review that employs a protocol to explore a broad topic area, sometimes to identify gaps in what is known

secondary source   a paper that reports on someone else's research study

self-determination   the freedom to make one's own decisions

simple random sampling   a sampling method where a random-number generator is used to select the required number of study participants from a population

skewed distribution   asymmetrical data distribution; when represented graphically, the curve has a longer tail at one end than the other

snowball sampling   a sampling method where current participants in a study recommend future potential participants

SQUIRE   a reporting standard for quality improvement studies

SRQR   a reporting standard for qualitative research

standard deviation   the square root of the variance, in essence correcting for the squaring of values that occurred in calculating the variance; it is nearly always used in preference to the variance

STARD   a reporting standard for diagnostic and prognostic studies

step-wedge cluster randomised controlled trial an experimental design in which groups of participants (clusters) begin the trial in the control condition and sequentially cross over to the intervention (experimental) condition.

stratified random sampling   a sampling method where the population is divided according to one or more characteristics and a random sample is drawn from each

STROBE   a reporting standard for observational studies

systematic review   a literature review that uses a structured question and search approach along with critical appraisal and quality analysis of studies

systematic sampling   a sampling method where participants are chosen not at random but according to a specific schedule

t-test   a statistical test used for comparing a continuous (ratio or interval) variable between two groups

thematic analysis   an interpretive process of organising qualitative data into themes

theme   a grouping of data containing similar meanings; it emerges through thematic analysis

theoretical sampling   a sampling technique used in grounded theory, involving sampling until the generated theory is complete

traditional narrative review   a subjective, non-critical review of the literature where included research is selected by the author

transferability   *see* fittingness or transferability

triangulation   the use of multiple methods or data sources that the researcher can verify and from which they can draw accurate conclusions

true experiment   *see* randomised controlled trial or true experiment

truncator   a symbol used at the end of part of a word in a database search to enable searching for all words that begin with the same letters

trustworthiness   the attribute of rigour in qualitative research

umbrella review   a systematic review of systematic reviews

validity of an instrument   the accuracy with which a research instrument or tool measures what it is supposed to measure

variable   any measured concept or characteristic that can vary in a study

variance   the average of the differences between each individual value and the mean

wildcard   a symbol used in place of a single letter to enable database searching for all variations of spelling

Index

abstract 14–15, 19, 81, 88, 136–137, 155, 165
Aboriginal and Torres Strait Islander peoples 104
action research *see* participatory action research
Advancing Research and Clinical Practice through Close Collaboration model 117
AGREE clinical guideline reporting standards 86, 165
analysis *see* data analysis
analysis of variance 56, 165
anonymity 104, 165
approval for research 32–33, 98–99; drugs or devices, research involving 32; ethics considerations 98–99; gatekeepers 33; institutions, from 32–33; randomised controlled trials, registration 32–33; sources 32–33
audience 37, 72, 137–140
Australian Code for the Responsible Conduct of Research *see* codes of conduct, research
Australian Commission on Safety and Quality in Health Care 3, 11
Australian and New Zealand Clinical Trials Registry 38, 151
Australian National Health and Medical Research Council (NHMRC) see National Health and Medical Research Council of Australia
Australian Research Council 154, 163
author guidelines 140–142
authorship 100, 141–142
autonomy 102, 165

beneficence 101–102, 165
bias 56, 84, 89, 165
bibliometric analysis 165
blinding 43, 165
blind review 142
Boolean operator 17–20, 165

CARE study reporting guidelines 86, 165
case-control design 42, 45–46, 165

case studies: barriers to handwashing 13; clinical research nurse 148; definition 165; effective handwashing 2; medication administration literature review 125; medication errors 112; person-centred care 26, 40, 61; publishing research 135; vital signs monitoring 78, 97
case study methodology 64
categorical/nominal data 47, 54, 56, 165
central tendency 52–54, 165; CHEERS 58; 165; mean 53–54, 169; median 53–54, 169; mode 53–54, 169
chi square 56, 165
citation 19, 79–80, 144
clinical audit xii, 115–116, 165
clinical doctorate 153, 165
clinical practice guidelines xii, 21–22, 86, 115, 165
clinical trials xii, 32–33, 38, 105, 149–152, 166
cluster randomised controlled trial *see* randomised controlled trials
codes of conduct, research 100, 109–110
coding 68–69, 166
coercion 104, 166
cohort design 42, 46–47, 166
Competencies for Registered Nurses 5
confidence intervals 54–56, 58, 166
confidentiality 82, 104, 160, 166
confirmability 71–72, 166
confounder, confounding 42–45, 56, 166
consent to research 34, 82, 102–104, 106–107, 158, 160; deferred or retrospective consent 103, 167; implied consent 103, 168; opt out consent 103, 169
CONSORT reporting standard 58, 86, 166
contamination 43, 166
content analysis xi, 68, 69–70, 166
continuity of care 122, 166
control group 42–44, 50
convenience sampling 50, 166
correlation 56, 166
correlational designs 42, 45–46, 49, 166

credibility xi, 7, 14–15, 71–72, 80–81, 139, 166; sources for checking 15

Critical Appraisal Skills Programme 85–86, 88, 166

critiquing research 78; abstract 81; author's reputation 79; conflicts of interest 84; data analysis 83; data collection 83; definition of critique 79, 166; ethical considerations 82; evaluation of journal quality 79–81; H-index 79, 144, 168; impact factor 80; importance of 79; interpretation of results 83; introduction and background 81; journal quality 14, 79–80; methodology 81–2; predatory journals 80, 140, 170; quartile ranking 80, 170; rapid reviews 93; research examples 84–85; research quality 79; scoping review 89–93; steps 78–84; structured critical literature review 85–86; study design 82; systematic review 87–89 (*see also* systematic review); title 79; tools for 85; umbrella reviews 93–94; *see also* literature review

cross-sectional design 45, 166

data: classification 34; definition 34, 166; qualitative 34; quantitative 34

data analysis 5, 36, 51, 166; common statistical tests and purposes 56; descriptive statistics 52–53; inferential statistics 53–54; normal distribution 52; qualitative research 68–70; quantitative research 51–56; realist evaluation 120–122; skewed distribution 52–53

data collection 4, 34–36; in action research 120; definition 34, 166; demographic 35; factors to consider 35; form of collection 35–36; interviews 35, 66; observation 35, 66; participants, sourcing 66–67; in qualitative research 65–66; in quantitative studies 50–51; in realist evaluation 121; research question and 35; sources of data 34–35; surveys 35, 51

data extraction 90, 92, 166

data immersion 68, 166

data saturation 67, 71, 72, 167

databases 9, 15–20; Boolean operator, use of 17, 19, 165; combining search terms 17; exploding search 18–19; focusing search 18–19; 'Full text available' 19; keyword searching 16; 'Limits' function 19; Medical Subject Headings (MeSH) 18–19, 169; MEDLINE 16–18; nursing and midwifery research articles 16; publication year 19; search terms 16;

specific phrase search 16; strategy for searching literature 20; synonyms, identification of 17; the tree 18; truncator symbol 17, 172; wildcard option 17, 172

Declaration of Helsinki 98, 167

deductive approach 41, 69, 167

dependability 71, 72, 167

dependent variable 47, 56, 57, 167

descriptive design, quantitative 45

descriptive statistics 51–52, 167; central tendency 52–53; dispersion 53; measurement scales and 54; when to use 53

discourse analysis 64, 65, 167

dispersion 52–53; definition 53, 167; frequency 53, 167; interquartile range 53, 168; percentile 53, 169; range 53, 170; standard deviation 53, 171; variance 53, 172

dissemination 5, 36–37, 135–145; conference 37, 136–138; definition 167; qualitative research reports 72; quantitative research reports 57–59; social networking sites 37; stakeholders 36–37; strategies 37; writing and publishing 141–145

double blinding 43

Enrolled Nurse Standards for Practice 5

EQUATOR Network 167; critiquing tools 85–86; reporting standards 59

ethics 4, 98–110, 135–136, 158, 160; anonymity 104, 165; autonomy 102, 165; beneficence 101–102, 165; clinical relationships 105; codes of conduct 100, 109–110; coercion 104, 166; confidentiality 82, 104, 160, 166; Declaration of Helsinki 98, 167; deferred or retrospective consent 103, 167; definition 167; discomfort 101; guidelines 97–98; harm 101; Human Research Ethics Committees (HRECs) 4, 32, 37, 72, 82, 98–99, 158, 160, 168; implied consent 103, 168; inconvenience 101; informed consent 34, 82, 102–104, 106–107, 158, 160, 168; international standards 98; internet and social media use 107; justice 105, 168; likelihood of adverse outcomes 101; non-maleficence 101–102, 169; Nuremberg Code 98, 169; opt out consent 103, 169; participant information statement 103; principles, development of 98; principles of ethical conduct of research 99–105;

privacy rights 104; reporting on ethical practices 105; research examples 106–107; research integrity 100, 170; research merit 99–100, 170; research procedures 32, 72, 82; research proposal 158; researchers, risk to 102; respect for persons 103–104; risk assessment 101–102; self-determination 103, 171
ethnography 64, 167
ethnomethodology 64, 167
evidence: definition 3, 167; finding 13–21; health professionals not using 3–4; implementation into practice 112–118; importance for health professional practice 2–4; judgement of 21–22; levels of 7–9 (*see also* hierarchy of evidence); relationship between research in nursing and midwifery and 3–7; sources of good evidence 13–15, 114–115; *see also* hierarchy of evidence
evidence-based practice 112–122; action research approach 64, 118–120; Advancing Research and Clinical Practice through Close Collaboration model 117; appraisal tools 85–86; barriers in 7; clinical audit 114–115; clinical practice guidelines 86, 113–114, 165; clinical practice, questioning 114, 115; definition 167; evaluation of practice change 118–122; evidence, identification of 112–118; hierarchy of evidence and 7–9; implementation of evidence into practice 115–116; implementation science 118, 168; implementation strategies 114–117; John Hopkins Nursing Evidence-Based Practice Model 117, 123; key requirement of nursing and midwifery 5–6; knowledge translation 112–113, 117, 168; midwifery, in 8; models 117–118; practice effectiveness 21; professional requirements for nurses and midwives 5–6; Promoting Action on Research 117; Implementation in Health Services (PARIHS) framework 117; rapid review 93–94, 170; realist evaluation 118, 120–122, 170; research examples 116, 119–120; sources of evidence for practice 114–115
experimental designs 41–45; intervention 41–42, 168; non-experimental designs and difference 41–42; quasi-experimental 44–45, 170; randomised controlled trial (RCT) (true experiment) 42–44, 170

fittingness/transferability 71, 167
focus groups 66, 120, 167
funding for clinical research 154

glossary 165–172
Google Scholar 15, 37, 88, 128–129
GRADE 9, 92–93, 167
grey literature 14, 88, 128, 167
grounded theory 63–64, 65, 67, 68, 81, 156, 168

h-index 79, 144, 168
hand hygiene 6, 9–10, 18–20
handsearching 88, 168
Health Research Authority UK 98
Health Research Council of New Zealand 98, 155
hierarchy of evidence 7–8, 21, 168; Joanna Briggs Institute (JBI) 21–22; randomised controlled trial (RCT) 42; systematic review (*see* systematic review)
honours degrees 152–153, 168
hospital-acquired infection 3, 10
Human Research Ethics Committees (HRECs) 32, 98–99, 101, 168; role 98–99
hypothesis 47, 156, 168; alternative 47; deductive approach 41; non-directional 47; null 47; realist evaluation 121

impact factor 80–81, 141, 168
implementation science 118, 168
independent variable 47, 54, 55, 56, 168
inductive approach 68, 168
inferential statistics 52, 53–54, 168; common statistical tests 56; confidence intervals 54–55, 166; probability 54, 170
information power 67, 168
integrative review 20, 28
International Academy of Nursing Editors (INANE) 80
International Committee on Publication Ethics (COPE) 80, 100
interpretive research 62, 168
intervention 16, 36, 41–42, 50, 87, 89, 91, 168
interviews 4, 35, 65–66, 82, 118, 120, 121, 157; interview schedule or guide 71, 82

Joanna Briggs Institute (JBI) 16, 89; approach to scoping reviews 91; critical appraisal tools 86; publication of evidence hierarchies 21; questions of 'meaningfulness' 21–22
John Hopkins Nursing Evidence-Based Practice Model 117, 123
journals 14, 79–80, 159; academic 14, 145; author 100, 141–142; editors 80; impact factor 80, 140, 167; peer review

14, 80, 142–143, 169; predatory 80,
170; publishing in 139–141; quality
79–80; quartile ranking 80, 170;
ranking 80; source of reported research
14; sources for checking credibility 15;
title of paper 79
justice 99, 105, 108, 168

keywords 9, 16–18, 88, 128, 129, 141;
combining 17–18; searching databases
16–18; spelling 17
knowledge translation 112–113, 117, 168

Likert scale 51, 168
literature review 4, 15, 87–94, 126; critiquing
81; definition 168; effective writing (*see*
writing literature reviews); emerging
approaches 93; narrative review 86;
purposes 4, 29, 126; rapid reviews 93;
research example of narrative review
127; research example of scoping review
126; research proposal 32, 155–162,
171; scoping review 86, 89–94, 171;
systematic review 87–89 (*see also*
systematic review); traditional narrative
review 86; types of 126; umbrella
reviews 93–94; use in research question
28–29; writing (*see* writing literature
reviews); *see also* critiquing research

Māori and Pacific Islander peoples 98, 104
masking 43, 168
mean 53–55, 169
measurement scales 47, 55; categorical/
nominal 47–48, 54, 56, 165; interval
48, 54–56, 58, 168; ordinal 48, 54,
169; ratio 48, 54, 56, 170
Medical Subject Headings (MeSH) 13, 18–20,
141, 145, 169; see also databases
MEDLINE 9, 16, 20, 88; barriers to
handwashing in nurses searches 13, 20
member checking 71, 149, 169
MeSH terms 20, 169; see also databases
methodology 14, 22, 29, 61, 64, 72, 81–83,
87, 169; qualitative research 29–31,
170; quantitative research 40–41;
definition 29, 169; *see also* mixed
methods research
midwife researcher 145, 148–150, 169
Midwife Standards for Practice 5
mixed methods research 30, 62, 169;
definition 169
mode 53–55, 165, 169

narrative review 86, 125–127, 129, 169, 171
National Health and Medical Research
Council of Australia 98, 109, 114, 123,

154, 163; ethics governance 98–99,
158, 160, 167–168; hierarchy of
evidence 7–9, 168
New Zealand National Ethics Advisory
Committee 98
NMBA see Nursing and Midwifery Board of
Australia
NMC see Nursing and Midwifery Council
non-directional hypothesis 47
non-experimental designs 41–42, 45;
case-control design 42, 45–46, 165;
cohort design 42, 45, 166; correlational
designs 42, 45, 49, 166; cross-sectional
design 40, 42, 45, 49, 137, 166;
descriptive 45, 167
non-maleficence 97, 99, 108, 169
normal distribution 52–54, 169
Nuremberg Code 98, 169
nurse researcher 148–149, 169
Nursing and Midwifery Board of Australia
5; Enrolled Nurse Standards for
Practice 5; Midwife Standards for
Practice 5; Registered Nurse Standards
for Practice 5; *see also* NMBA
Nursing and Midwifery Council 5; Standards
of Proficiency for Midwives 6;
Standards of Proficiency for Registered
Nurses 5; *see also* NMC

observation 4, 35, 41, 57, 65–66, 71–72,
106, 118–121, 131, 157, 169; data
collection method 4, 35, 41, 65, 66, 72,
120–121, 169; ethical issues 106; see
also participant observation
Office for Human Research Protections 98
ordinal data 48, 54, 169

paradigm 29, 62, 72, 169
participatory action research 118–120, 169
peer review 14, 80, 142, 169
phenomenology 63–65, 81, 119, 156, 160, 169
photovoice 66, 170
PICO 16, 87–88, 91, 170
PICOS 87
PICOT 87
population 16, 33, 35, 49–50, 52–55, 64, 66,
71, 83, 87, 170–171
practice effectiveness 21
practice guidelines *see* clinical practice
guidelines
presentation skills 135–139, 145
primary source 81, 125, 129, 159, 170
probability 49–50, 54, 169; sampling methods
49, 169
Promoting Action on Research Implementation
in Health Services (PARIHS)
framework 117

publication 79–80, 100, 136, 139, 143–145, 165–169
publishing 80, 139, 144–145

qualitative research 29–31, 62–68, 70–73, 83, 86, 156, 158, 167–172; action research 62, 64, 66, 113, 118–120, 122, 166, 169; approaches 29, 62; audit trail 72; case study 64, 165; coding 68, 166; confirmability 71–72, 166; content analysis 68–70, 166; credibility 71–72, 166; data analysis in 68–69; data collection 65–66, 167; data immersion 68, 166; data saturation 67, 71–72, 167; definition 170; dependability 71–72, 167; descriptive 63, 65, 67, 70, 165, 67; discourse analysis 64–65, 167; ethnography 64, 167; ethnomethodology 64, 167; fittingness 71, 167; focus groups 66, 121, 151, 167; grounded theory 63–65, 67, 168; historical approach 64, 168; immersion 68, 166; inductive approach 68, 168; interpretive 62, 168, 171; interviews 4, 8, 35, 63, 65–67, 69–72, 82–83, 101–102, 118–121, 154, 158, 160–161, 167–168; member checking 71, 169; methodology 63–65, 72, 81–83, 87, 120, 169; narrative research 64, 169; nursing and midwifery, common approaches in 63–64; paradigms 62, 169; participant observation 66, 169; participatory research 66, 169; person-centred care, exploring 30, 65, 67, 69–70; phenomenology 63–64, 160, 169–170; photovoice 66, 170; planning 67; quality and rigour strategies 71–72; quantitative research and, differences 29–31; realities 62; reporting findings 72; research question, developing 64–65; sampling 66–68; sourcing research participants 66–68; steps in undertaking 64–70; suitable questions for 64–65; surveys 66; thematic analysis 68–69; themes 68–69; transferability 71–72, 167, 171; triangulation 71, 171
quality patient care 3–4
quantitative research 29–31, 40–41, 170; aims of 40–41; basis of 40–41; cause-and-effect relationships 41–42, 170; comparison of designs 42, 46; data analysis 51–56; data collection 50–51; deductive approach 41, 167; definition 41, 170; descriptive quantitative design 42, 45–46, 50–51, 167; designs 41–46; experimental designs 41–45

(see also experimental designs); hypothesis 47, 57, 156, 167–168; measurement 29, 44, 47, 52–57; non-experimental designs 41–42, 45 (*see also* non-experimental designs); objectivity 41; operationalising concepts 46; qualitative research and, differences 29–31; reliability 56–58; reporting findings 57–59; reporting standards 58–59; research question, developing 64–65; research rigour 56–57; sampling, approaches to 49–50; suitable questions for 30; validity 56–57, 172; variable 41, 47–48, 52–53, 54–56
quartile ranking 80, 170
quasi-experimental designs 44–45, 170; control group 44; evidence hierarchy, place in 45; person-centred care example 48; pre-post test 44, 170; two-group non-randomised non-parallel design 44
quota sampling 50, 170

randomised controlled trials (RCTs) 9, 32, 170; blinding 43, 165; cluster randomised controlled trial 43–44, 166; confounder 42–44, 166; contamination 43, 166; control group 42–44, 50, 170; disadvantages 43; elements of 42; intervention 42, 168; masking 43, 168; random allocation 42; stratified randomisation 43, 171; step-wedge randomised controlled trial 43–44, 171; two-group parallel RCT 42–43
rapid review 93–94, 170
ratio data 170
realist evaluation 118, 120–122, 170; concepts 120; context 120; context mechanism outcome pattern configuration (CMOC) 120; cycle of 120–121; data analysis 121; data collection 121; hypothesis 121; mechanism 120; midwifery practice 122; nursing practice 121; outcome patterns 120; research example 121–122; theory testing 121
Registered Nurse Standards for Practice 5
regression 56–58, 170
reliability 170
reporting standards 58; CARE 86, 165; CONSORT 58, 86, 166; EQUATOR Network 59, 85–86, 167; PRISMA 86, 89; SQUIRE 58, 86, 171; SRQR 86, 171; STARD 58, 171; STROBE 58, 171
research: aim 28–29, 170; barriers in evidence-based nursing practice 7;

critique of study (*see* critiquing research); ethics (*see* ethics); evidence-based practice in midwifery 8; hand hygiene practices 9–10; ideas for (*see* research question); integrity 100, 170; levels of evidence (*see* evidence); merit 99–100, 170; nurses and midwives as users of 5–6, 20–21; relationship between evidence and 3–4; study designs 21–22

research midwife 149, 171

research nurse 148–149, 171

research participants: confidentiality 82, 104, 160, 166; deferred or retrospective consent 103, 167, 171; ethical treatment of (*see* ethics); exclusion criteria 34, 167; implied consent 103–104, 168; inclusion criteria 168; informed consent 102–104, 160, 168; interviews 35, 65–66, 69–70, 168; Likert scale 51, 168; observation 65–66, 169; opt out consent 103, 169; population 33, 35, 49–50, 53, 66, 170–171; privacy 104; recruitment 34, 105; sample 33–35, 49–50, 171; sampling 66–68, 166, 169–171; selecting 33–34, 171; sourcing 66; vulnerability 98

research pathways for nurses and midwives: clinical doctorate 153, 166; clinical trial nurse 149; clinical trials 149–150, 166, 171; Doctor of Philosophy 153, 159; education 152–154; evidence generator 149; funding 154–155; honours degrees 152–153, 168; midwife researcher 145, 148–150, 169; nurse researcher 148–149, 169; professional doctorates 153; research degree 152, 154, 170; research midwife 149, 171; research nurse 148–149, 171; research proposal 32, 155–162, 171

research process 4, 10, 26, 32–38, 41, 171; approach, selection of 32; approval to undertake 32; communication of findings 33, 36, 136–144; data analysis 5, 36, 51–53, 68–69, 166; data collection 4, 35, 47, 51, 66, 68, 71, 83, 120–121, 157, 166; definition 171; ethical approval 4, 99, 167; interpretation of findings 36, 71, 83, 166; methodology 14, 22, 29, 61, 64, 72, 8–83, 87, 169; mixed methods approach 21, 30–31, 62, 169; paradigm 29, 62, 72, 169; participants, selecting 33–34, 171; presenting findings 136–144; publishing findings 139–144; qualitative approach 21, 30,

36, 38, 63–64; quantitative approach 30, 33, 40–41, 46, 61; reporting (*see* dissemination); research proposal, writing 32, 155–162; steps in 4

research proposal 32, 155–162, 171 abstract 155; additional hints for writing 161–162; appendices 159; budget and resources 158; data collection 157; data management and analysis 157; definition 171; dissemination plan 159; ethical considerations 158; example of nursing research 159–161; instruments 157; introduction and background 155; literature review 156; participants 157; references 159; research design 156; research methods 157; research problem, aim and question 156; research team 159; study significance 156; theoretical framework 156; timeline 158; title 155; tools of data collection 157; writing 32, 155–162

research question: broad topic of interest 27; definition 171; developing in qualitative approach 64–65; developing in quantitative approach 46–47; person-centred care example 65, 67; research aim and 27; research approach and 46–47, 64–67

research rigour 56–59, 72; bias 56, 58–59, 84, 165; reliability 56–57, 58, 59, 170; trustworthiness 72, 172; validity 56–59, 172

researchers: ethical responsibilities (*see* ethics); nurses and midwives as 148–152

reviews: integrative 20, 28; narrative 86, 94, 127, 129, 169; rapid 93–94, 141, 170; scoping 85–86, 89, 91–94, 120, 126–127, 151, 171; systematic 7, 9–10, 15–16, 21, 79, 84, 86–91, 132, 170–171; umbrella 28, 93, 94, 172

sample 33–35, 49–50, 171

sample size 34, 43, 49–50, 58, 67, 100, 168, 170

sampling: cluster random 50, 166; convenience 50, 166; non-probability 50, 169; power of study 50, 67, 168, 170; probability 50, 54, 169, 170; purposive 50, 66–67, 170; quota 50, 170; sample size and 49–50; simple random 49, 171; snowball 67, 160, 171; stratified random 49, 171; systematic 50, 171; theoretical 67, 171

scoping review 86, 89–94, 171; concept 91–92; context 91–92; definition 171; Joanna Briggs Institute approach 91; protocol,

developing 92; research example
    92–93, 126–127, 151–152; types of
    participants 91–92; *see also* literature
    review
search engines 15, 128–129
search terms 16, 88
secondary sources 129
single blinding 43
skewed distribution 52–54, 171
social media use 144, 159; nursing and
    midwifery research, in 107–108
SQUIRE reporting standard 58, 86, 171
SRQR reporting standard 86, 171
standard deviation 53–54, 167, 171
Standards of Clinical & Cultural Competence
    & Conduct 5
Standards of Proficiency for Midwives 6
Standards of Proficiency for Registered Nurses 5
STARD reporting standard 58, 171
statistical tests: analysis of variance 56, 165;
    chi square 56, 165; correlation 56, 166;
    regression 56–58, 170; t-test 56, 171
STROBE reporting standard 58, 86, 171
survey 50–51, 57, 66, 85, 102, 107; ethical
    issues 107; qualitative research 66;
    quantitative research 50–51; research
    example 85
systematic review 9–10; conduct of search
    88–89; definition 9, 171; extraction
    and synthesis of data 89; flow chart
    of search 89–90; hand hygiene, of
    10; inclusion criteria 88; key aspects
    (PICO) 87; PICO 87, 170; protocol
    development 88, 171; quality appraisal
    tools 88; quality of studies 88; research
    example 91; retrieved studies, selection
    of 89–90; review protocol, developing
    88; review question, developing 87;
    search strategy 88

t-test 56, 171
Te Kaunihera Tapuhi o Aotearoa/Nursing
    Council of New Zealand 5;
    Competencies for Registered Nurses 5

Te Tatau o te Whare Kahu/Midwifery Council
    5; Standards of Clinical & Cultural
    Competence & Conduct 5
textbooks 14–15, 129
thematic analysis 68–69, 171
trial registries 33
triangulation 71, 171; data source 71;
    investigator 71; method 71; theory 71
true experiments *see* randomised controlled
    trials (RCTs)
truncator 88, 129, 172; *see also* databases
two-group non-randomised non-parallel
    design 44

UK National Institute for Health and Care
    Research 114, 154
umbrella review 28, 93, 94, 172

validity 56–57; external 56, 89, 167;
    instrument, of 172; internal 56, 168
variable 41, 47–48, 50, 52–56; dependent
    47, 167; independent 47, 168;
    measurement of 47, 50; values 47–48,
    52–56

wildcard 17, 172; option for database searches
    17, 172
World Health Organization 3, 32–33; practice
    guidelines for hand hygiene 3
writing literature reviews 128–132;
    clarification of question 128;
    conclusion 130; definition of
    literature review 125–126, 168; direct
    quotations 131, 167; introduction 130;
    paraphrasing 130–131, 169; planning
    130; primary sources 129; purposes
    of literature reviews 126; reading and
    critiquing 129; research example of
    systematic review 132; review body
    130; searching for literature 128–129;
    secondary sources 128–129; selection
    of literature to include 129; sources of
    literature 129; synthesising ideas 130;
    types of literature reviews 126

Taylor & Francis eBooks

www.taylorfrancis.com

A single destination for eBooks from Taylor & Francis
with increased functionality and an improved user
experience to meet the needs of our customers.

90,000+ eBooks of award-winning academic content in
Humanities, Social Science, Science, Technology, Engineering,
and Medical written by a global network of editors and authors.

TAYLOR & FRANCIS EBOOKS OFFERS:

A streamlined
experience for
our library
customers

A single point
of discovery
for all of our
eBook content

Improved
search and
discovery of
content at both
book and
chapter level

REQUEST A FREE TRIAL
support@taylorfrancis.com

 Routledge
Taylor & Francis Group

 CRC Press
Taylor & Francis Group

Printed in the United States
by Baker & Taylor Publisher Services